The Viral Network

EXPERTISE

**CULTURES AND
TECHNOLOGIES
OF KNOWLEDGE**

EDITED BY DOMINIC BOYER

A list of titles in this series is available at www.cornellpress.cornell.edu.

THE VIRAL NETWORK

A Pathography of the H1N1 Influenza Pandemic

THERESA MacPHAIL

CORNELL UNIVERSITY PRESS
ITHACA AND LONDON

First published 2014 by Cornell University Press
First printing, Cornell Paperbacks, 2014
Printed in the United States of America

Library of Congress Cataloging-in-Publication Data

MacPhail, Theresa, 1972– author.
    The viral network : a pathography of the H1N1 influenza pandemic /
Theresa MacPhail.
        pages cm. — (Expertise)
    Includes bibliographical references (p.   ).
    ISBN 978-0-8014-5240-6 (cloth : alk. paper)
    ISBN 978-0-8014-7983-0 (pbk. : alk. paper)
    1. H1N1 influenza. 2. Epidemics—Social aspects. 3. Public health—
Social aspects. 4. Medical anthropology. I. Title.
    RA644.I6M33   2014
    614.5'18—dc23   2014025187

Cornell University Press strives to use environmentally responsible
suppliers and materials to the fullest extent possible in the publishing
of its books. Such materials include vegetable-based, low-VOC inks
and acid-free papers that are recycled, totally chlorine-free, or partly
composed of nonwood fibers. For further information, visit our
website at www.cornellpress.cornell.edu.

Cloth printing   10 9 8 7 6 5 4 3 2 1
Paperback printing   10 9 8 7 6 5 4 3 2 1

Contents

Acknowledgments

Writing an acknowledgments section is a very daunting task. So many individuals and institutions are responsible for the production of this book that I am at a loss as to where to begin my thanks. However, this project would not have been possible at all without the generosity of the epidemiologists and scientists who allowed me to observe them, to participate in their day-to-day lives, to interview them, to learn their lab techniques, and to share their bevy of knowledge and experience with me. My sincerest gratitude goes out to them—both for letting me work with them and, more importantly, for their tireless efforts to keep all of us safer. The men and women who work in public health are, I can attest, some of the most dedicated, smart, unflagging, and overworked people on this planet. If it weren't for them, we'd all be a lot sicker. Special thanks to Rohit Chitale, Kira Christian, Mike Schwartz, Fred Leung, and most importantly, Ray Arthur.

I would also like to extend a special thanks to Chris Ansell and Ann Keller at the University of California, Berkeley, who supported part of this research with their National Science Foundation grant. It was under their auspices that I began this research and I will be forever indebted to both of them for their insights, guidance, and support. As well, I'd like to extend thanks to the interdisciplinary team of researchers that worked together to collect data for the project: Erik Baaskeslov, Sahai Burrowes, and Mark Hunter. Especially Mark, who provided me with the amazing timeline that appears in the introduction to this book.

While in California, I was fortunate to have some excellent mentors and readers of my work: the indefatigable Vincanne Adams, Cori Hayden, Kevin O'Brien, Lawrence Cohen, Sharon Kaufman, Charles Briggs, and Nancy Scheper-Hughes. At New York University, I was privileged to learn strategies for success from Robin Nagle, Robert Dimit, Rayna Rapp, and Emily Martin. My writing here would not have progressed as smoothly without them. I also want to thank my compatriots at New York University who provided me with happy hours, movies, conversation, laughter, and all the miscellaneous distractions so crucial to good thinking: Mario Caro, Alan Itkin, Georgia Lowe, Steve Moga, and Amber Musser. The Ph.D. candidates in my two-week intensive writing workshops at NYU were often an invaluable source of inspiration; my gratitude to Laurie Benton, Kathy Talvecchia, and Anne Bernadette-Waters for giving me the opportunity to mentor these beginning scholars as I finished writing this book.

Institutional support for both my research and my writing was provided by the University of California, Berkeley, and the D. Kim Foundation. A version of chapter 5 was published as "A Predictable Unpredictability: The 2009 H1N1 Pandemic and the Concept of 'Strategic Uncertainty' within Global Public Health," *Behemoth* 3 (3): 55–77.

A very special thanks must go to Xin Liu, who not only taught me how to ask the right questions, but counseled that answers are always to be found while reading another book, doing more research, and writing. Another special thanks to Tim Choy, who provided me with the solidarity and insights that could only come from a fellow Hong Kong scholar. His notes on my Hong Kong chapters made all the difference. Andrew Lakoff also could not have been more helpful, nor a better champion for my work. And then, of course, there is the person who first started me on my anthropological wanderings: Stefan Helmreich. Without him, I'd probably still be a journalist. Infinite gratitude is due my series editor, Dominic Boyer, without whom this book would be a pale shadow of itself. Dominic, in sum, coached and pestered and encouraged me into being a far better scholar and academic writer. I thank him for encouraging me to be both bold and more concise. And thanks, too, to editor Peter Potter, who recognized the early potential of this project.

And finally, the personal thanks. To Eric Plemons, the best writing partner anyone has ever had, a "thank you" doesn't even begin to cover it. My brilliant friend Matt Lawlor, scientist extraordinaire, took the time to painstakingly check my explanations of the virus's biology. I owe him many libations. To the wonderful women of the Science and Technology Studies writing group: Jade Sasser, Martine Lappe, Katie Hasson, Rachel Washburn. To Sam Howard-Spink, for coffee and jelly bean breaks. To my University of California, Berkeley friends, who continue to provide me with inspiration, but especially: James Battle, Shana Harris, Andy Hao, Katie Hendy, Liz Kelley, Kelly Knight, Xochitl Marsilli Vargas, Amelia Moore, Suepattra May Slater, and Emily Wilcox. To my chosen family, without whom I could do nothing well: Pat, Cara, Rebecca, Robin, Mark, Annika, Jan Fak, Glen, Jon, Martha, Jason, Andrea, and Hugh. To Sloan, a special thank you for putting up with me during fieldwork and my dissertation process, and for reminding me on a weekly basis that I am a solid writer. I hope I can return the favor someday.

And finally, to Kyle Levenick, for showing me how to say "yes" more often in the long-form improvisation that is life.

Abbreviations

BSL-2	Biosafety Level 2
CDC	United States Centers for Disease Control
CHP	Centre for Health Protection (Hong Kong)
CPE	Cytopathic effect
DNA	Deoxyribonucleic acid
ENDS	Emergent Networks, Distributed Sensemaking project
GISN	Global Influenza Surveillance Network
GISRS	Global Influenza Surveillance and Response System
GDDOC	Global Disease Detection Operations Center (CDC)
HA	Hemagglutinin
HPAI	High Pathogenic Avian Influenza
ILI	Influenza-like illness
LPAI	Low Pathogenic Avian Influenza
MDCK cells	Madin-Darby Canine Kidney cells
NA	Neuraminidase
NIH	National Institutes of Health

PAHO   Pan American Health Organization, a regional office of
           the WHO
PCR   Polymerase chain reaction
RNA   Ribonucleic acid
SAR   Special Administrative Region (Hong Kong)
SARS   Severe Acute Respiratory Syndrome
SME   Subject matter expert
$TCID_{50}$ 50 percent tissue culture infective dose
WHO   World Health Organization

THE VIRAL NETWORK

Prologue to a Pathography

Learning to Cover Your Mouth

In January 2004, I was sitting on the ferry from Jiangmen to Hong Kong, returning from a sightseeing holiday in Guangdong Province. The region was still reeling from the 2003 SARS epidemic, and television commercials urged citizens to be "vigilant and prepared" against its possible recurrence in the spring. In addition to the SARS virus, another recent outbreak of the avian influenza virus H5N1 in China's southern neighbor, Vietnam, had caused a mounting fear of a future "bird flu" pandemic. Worry over virus outbreaks was spreading across Southeast Asia faster than the viruses themselves. As I sat on the ferry, wedged between two Chinese men and listening to the seasonal coughs and sneezes all around me, I felt for the first time a spark of dread myself. Viruses were very much on my mind, but especially influenza.

In Hong Kong, "the flu" seemed to be everywhere I looked. It lurked in the famed bird market in Kowloon, among the rows of exotic parakeets,

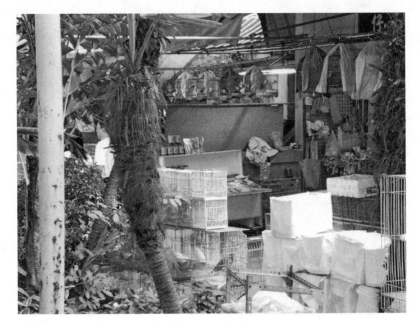

Figure 1. Kowloon's bird market, Hong Kong.

song birds, and canaries for sale as prized pets. It nested in the rows and rows of fresh chicken stalls on the lower level of the huge, multistory food market in Central District. I saw shadows of it in the enormous shuttered abattoir deep in the heart of Kowloon. Face masks on bus passengers reminded me of it. Posters hung up around Hong Kong—on buses, in hotel lobbies, all along the Midlevels escalator—reflected the government and the medical community's concern, displaying easy-to-follow instructions about how to avoid catching the disease by coming into contact with live chickens, ducks, or other birds and their feces. During intermittent outbreaks of H5N1, the US Consulate in Hong Kong emailed bulletins to its citizens detailing how to minimize risk and what the US government was doing about avian influenza. By the time I left China in late 2006, avian flu had become the new watchword of global disease prevention, on the lips of WHO members and nighttime news anchors as much local populations.

On that crowded ferry trip from Jiangmen, I rediscovered that I was susceptible. Not only in the immunological, or bodily, sense of the word, but in the more ideological sense, or mentally and emotionally. The influenza virus might eventually make its way into my upper respiratory tract, but it had already infected my thinking. And from even a cursory examination of local and international newspaper reports on H5N1, or during simple conversations with other passengers on the ferry, I knew I was not alone in my anxiety. As we heeded the advice to wash our hands frequently, to keep a polite social distance from each other, and to cover our noses and mouths when we coughed or sneezed, we remained afraid that merely knowing the dangers of influenza and taking simple precautionary measures to control its spread would not be enough to protect us.

The growing specter of a global pandemic of influenza—specifically, one more generically referred to in both public health circles and in the popular press as being caused by avian influenza or "bird flu" or H5N1—spurred a fascination or myopia in policy circles as much as in the media. Over a decade of pandemic planning had focused almost exclusively upon H5N1 and had ultimately left public health institutions at the local, national and international levels largely unprepared for a pandemic of a milder strain of influenza—in this case, the "swine flu," the novel H1N1 influenza outbreak that occurred in the early spring of 2009. The historical planning emphasis on "bird flu," as one public health official suggested during a closed conference on H1N1 held in the summer of 2009, had unintentionally created a large amount of uncertainty about how to respond to any other, milder type of infectious disease threat. The public health community, it seemed, had become too engrossed by the possibility of bird flu coming out of Asia to pay much attention to the early warning signs of a late-season outbreak of an influenza-like illness in Mexico.

Yet many of the same epidemiologists and virologists who expressed frustration with the limitations of pandemic plans modeled on H5N1 also noted that the planning efforts themselves had been integral to building and strengthening relationships among far-flung colleagues, national public health agencies, and international health institutions. The flu experts I worked with or interviewed throughout the 2009 pandemic believed that the resultant networks and personal bonds had positively affected the overall speed and efficiency of the global public health response to H1N1. Planning, then, was often conceptualized as a double-edged sword.

Part of the problem with preparing for a deadlier outbreak, epidemiologists often explained to me, was that most local and national flu plans had unintentionally constrained the range of possible actions throughout the 2009 pandemic. What might be effective procedures during a terrifying, deadly outbreak might not be as helpful during a moderately severe or milder one. As one epidemiologist aptly parsed it, once public health experts had collectively "flipped the switch" on the global pandemic response to the H1N1 influenza virus, individual agencies were then unable to easily retool, reconfigure, or shut down local response actions as the situation continued to develop. Most responders felt increasingly locked in to protocols that were modeled on an outbreak of a significantly more pathogenic influenza virus. By the late fall of 2009, and despite the fact that most experts had concluded that H1N1 was a much milder threat than had been originally anticipated, public health agencies remained tied into practices—such as case counting—that many epidemiologists felt were virtually useless. Such practices were not only time-consuming but diverted manpower away from the more routine tasks of detecting and responding to other, potentially more serious, health threats.

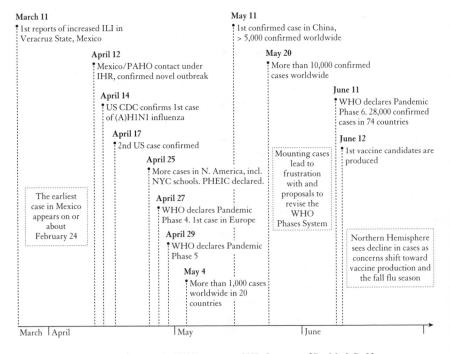

Figure 2. Key early events in H1N1 response, 2009. Courtesy of Dr. Mark D. Hunter.

This friction between a projected pandemic based on models and forecasting and the "real-time" events that took place throughout 2009 and into 2010 led to a palpable tension between what an epidemiologist or virologist might state openly in the media or in a government report and what he might say freely or "off the record" among his colleagues or to people who had access to similar contextual information related to local or regional outbreaks (for more on the role of context, see chapter 6). By late 2009, the fact that the pandemic was all but over had become an open secret—albeit one that was only circulated within public health agencies or among trusted partners in the global public health network. In other words, learning to "cover your mouth" during an influenza pandemic meant learning which stories might be told openly and which ones should only be shared within trusted circles. Much like the advice experts dispensed about the need to cover one's mouth throughout the flu season, knowing how to discern or relay useful information or when to exchange gut feelings or "best guesses" during the pandemic was simply part of learning how to be "polite" within cultures of expertise.

This book is, in its most basic form, a compendium of some of the fragmented and partial accounts of the 2009 H1N1 pandemic. It is a story of other people's stories, a narrative of other narratives. Ultimately, then, this book is written as a pathography of global public health's experience with "having the flu."

On Pathography

Pathography—a term more typically associated with medicine, or with literature describing a retrospective or biographical study of the effects of an illness or disease on individuals or communities—is defined here as the combination of historical, biological, social, individual, political, economic, and cultural narratives of a disease or its outbreak, in this case the 2009 H1N1 pandemic. As such, it is inherently multisited and embedded in multiple time frames at once. For my purposes, however, the term pathography refers not only to an end product or the narratives constructed within these pages, but also to a methodology for analyzing the various public health responses to the recent 2009 H1N1 influenza pandemic. A pathography is a method for coming to terms with the myriad effects, both positive and negative, on our worlds of any crisis, chronic illness, or contagious disease.[1]

By this definition, then, the concept of pathography acts as an extension of traditional ethnography. Ethnography relies upon participant observation as its grounding methodology; so does pathography. Both depend for their insights not only on the participant observation of the ethnographer, but on a variety of other equally important sources and activities: the reading of historical texts, as well as newspaper and other media accounts; the interpretation of photographs and charts; the unpacking of hearsay and gossip; the analysis of official reports, conference calls, and meetings; and the act of consulting or helping to produce policy. Yet in comparison, pathography takes a disease, illness, or crisis—and its attendant stories—as its grounding object. A pathography is not only a description of events, or a combination of scientific fieldwork and intuitive understanding, but an attempt to produce a type of metanarrative about crisis or disease in a specific time, place, and setting.

An important aside here on metanarratives, or, a brief examination of why I want to self-consciously situate pathography as an effort to partially rehabilitate the concept of grand narratives (Lyotard 1984). In a post-postmodern world, is the telling of smaller or fragmented stories the only possible response to what many see as the hegemonic and dangerous side of metanarratives? At the start of the twenty-first century, are grand narratives either impossible or dangerous to construct? I don't think so. Pathography is necessarily fragmented—it recounts and examines various pieces of a larger story; but those fragments are necessarily connected to form a larger, "grander" narrative— through their combination and recombination we can learn something not only about "what happened," but something about ourselves and the world. In my definition, then, pathography is a shameless metanarrative As a piece of writing, it is about trying to say something about the universal through an interweaving of the particular.

Pathography is a product of the shift in anthropology's object of study in the twenty-first century and the escalating trend in the social sciences writ large toward the interdisciplinary. Clearly, pathography and ethnography are similar, both as methods and as end products. But in addition to a pathography being centered on adverse things and events, there is one other unmistakable and crucial distinction between them: a pathography takes seriously the notion that nonhuman actors—here the disease or disease organism itself—have a certain type of nontrivial agency in the world. Viruses in this pathography are informants as well as biological entities at the center of a dynamic scientific research program and at the heart of robust international pandemic prevention policies and planning. In other words, the 2009 H1N1 Influenza A virus in this book is a subject (in both meanings of the term) as much as it is an object. The influenza virus in this book is not merely a trope for global public health, or our information-centric times, or an increasingly interconnected world; instead, I argue that influenza has partially constructed—and continues to shape—the contours of that world.

Depicting influenza viruses as key informants here is tied up with far larger political and epistemological questions concerning the agential relationships between human and nonhuman actors (Hayden 2003, Helmreich 2009, Mitchell 2002). The H1N1 and H5N1 viruses are, so to speak, my dual guides throughout this pathography. I follow them as a forensic journalist would track a money trail or trace email messages. I encounter them in the field and examine them under microscopes. I do not merely observe viruses, I try to "be with" them as they help to build and flow through networks of scientific expertise. As with the virologists and epidemiologists at the core of this pathography, my own knowledge production, expertise, and passions are inextricably entangled in a shifting, evolving mess of viral RNA. Make no mistake; viruses are always at the heart of the multilayered, multiscaled story that is about to unfold.

The way this book is written is—in point of fact—part of its overall argument. In order to understand any pandemic or infectious disease outbreak, one must attempt to look at its various biological, social, political, and historical narratives concurrently. The biggest challenge in writing a pathography of unfolding events, in this case the "swine flu" or H1N1 outbreaks of 2009, is to make sense out of the various and still emerging accounts of those events. How can we write about something as it happens? How can we tell the story of a story as it unfolds? To make matters even more difficult, I was inside the story of H1N1 from the beginning of the so-called second wave of the outbreak; my research began *in medias res*, not *ex post facto*. The immediate result of this submersion in the public health landscape during the H1N1 pandemic has been that perspective, so to speak, has consistently been hard to come by. Rather than endeavor to write a strictly linear "story" of the pandemic, or an ethnography, then, in this book I attempt to re-create and analyze the various stories—historical, scientific, global, political, popular, and personal—about what is commonly referred to as "the flu."

The Biological Uniqueness of Viruses

Why viruses? What is it about these invisible entities that fascinates, terrifies, and obsesses us? That compels us to spend billions of dollars researching, studying, and tracking them globally? Some microbes are deadly, it's true, and their effects on humans and animals can be truly horrific and costly, but our collective and arguably sensible quest for better health is not necessarily the only reason viruses have become the center of such a vast program of global surveillance and scientific research. To begin to understand how influenza viruses have become so mesmerizing, we first need to unpack their unique biology.

To start, viruses really are "special." They are exceptional in that they cannot replicate, or make copies of themselves, outside of a host cell. Unlike bacteria and other cellular organisms, viruses cannot perform most of their biological functions alone. They must invade and "hijack" a cell's mechanisms in order to manufacture the proteins necessary for their replication. Because of this, viruses are typically conceptualized as lying somewhere on a spectrum between living and nonliving things. They are liminal objects with some of the properties of "life" and yet cannot be considered fully "alive" while outside of a permissive host. Viruses are, in essence, simply packets of pure information—genetic material in the form of either DNA or RNA, though RNA viruses are far more common—within an encasement of protein. They are the single most common and plenteous organism on our planet. Viruses can be found almost everywhere: in the tundra of the Arctic, at the bottom of the sea floor, in the soil, and inside almost every other living creature. Viruses are even in our own genetic makeup; so-called "junk DNA" in the human genome is riddled with viral remnants, as evidence either of past infections or of a long-standing symbiotic partnership (depending on who you ask). And while the origin of viruses remains unclear, speculation about them is rife. Either viruses evolved along with bacteria and other single-cell organisms in the primordial sea, or they were the progenitors of bacteria and other single-cell organisms, or they are simply genetic material that "escaped" from single-cell organisms millions of years ago. Inconsequential to which origin story might be correct, viruses are evidently hardy survivors. Their famed ability to evolve quickly, evading immune systems and other means of eradicating them, inspires not only fear but awe. Virologists marvel at viruses' innate talent for innovation, their speed of information exchange, their diversity, their ability to adapt and survive under conditions that would cripple or kill other organisms.

Influenza A, B, and C viruses are part of a small family of RNA viruses called Orthomyxoviridae (which roughly translates to "straight mucus"). Influenza viruses produce a week-long illness and typically attack the upper respiratory system (thus making the "mucus" part of their Greek nomenclature above particularly apropos), although the virus can and often does spread to other areas of the body such as the intestinal tract. At the flu's onset, symptoms can include fever, headache, body aches, fatigue, sneezing, coughing, and sore throat. Periodically, and with alarming regularity, more severe influenza pandemics sweep the globe; three such pandemics occurred in the last century alone, in 1918 (the deadliest on record), 1957, and 1968. The H1N1 pandemic in 2009, though mild, was the first of the new century, but it will likely not be the last.

Each influenza virus contains a genome made up of eight individual gene segments; not a lot of genetic information, especially considering how much damage they can do once inside a host. All are able to infect humans and certain animals (including birds, pigs, horses, dogs, cats, ferrets, and seals), but Influenza A and B viruses are the most common culprits in human infections and normal seasonal pandemics.[2] Of the three virus genera, Influenza A is of most concern to virologists and epidemiologists and will be the focus of this pathography. Mutation is a virus's method of evolution and Influenza A is particularly good at it. RNA viruses such as Influenza A regularly mutate as they replicate (a process known as antigenetic drift), but can also swap entire genetic segments with other viruses inside a host (a process known as antigenetic shift).

Virologists who study influenza are particularly interested in any genetic changes in regions of the virus's genome that may affect the composition of the surface proteins of the virus, or its antigens. Antigens are substances that provoke a response by the host's immune system, which then produces antibodies to fight off infection. When the host's immune system does not recognize novel antigens, such as those produced by antigenetic shift, it is slower to protect against illness—which can result in a more debilitating infection.

The antigens of importance to virologists who study Influenza A are hem-agglutinin (HA) and neuraminidase (NA), spike-like protuberances on the surface of the influenza virus. Influenza A viruses are typed and named by their H and N numbers, each number representing a different protein sub-type.[3] Routine surveillance of influenza viruses focuses on any incremental changes or dramatic shifts in genetic makeup that directly influence the HA and NA proteins (I examine the practice of surveillance and genetic sequencing further in chapter 1). Most virologists see the HA and NA anti-gens as key[4] to the influenza virus's capacity to spread quickly and to cause more serious—and sometimes deadly—variants of the flu.

In addition to subtype, Avian Influenza A viruses are also categorized by how pathogenic, or able to cause disease, they are. Pathogenicity is char-acterized by a virus's molecular makeup (tracked via genetic sequencing and the production of phylogenetic, or evolutionary, trees) and its ability to affect serious illness in its host species—birds—under either experimental or actual conditions. A "low path" or Low Pathogenic Avian Influenza (LPAI) virus is one that affects only mild disease in ducks, chickens, or geese. A "high-path" or Highly Pathogenic Avian Influenza (HPAI) virus causes a severe, and often lethal, illness in its avian hosts. HPAI viruses are considered to be of serious potential threat to humans; when such a virus makes the occasional "jump" from its host species into a human host, the resulting infection is usually severe and fatal. While such infections remain rare (and largely concentrated in those who come into daily close contact with poultry), the worry is that such a "rogue" HPAI virus will meet a "regular" influenza virus in its human (or swine) host, swap genetic mate-rial, and combine to produce a super virus—one easily spread from human to human and capable of causing a lethal pandemic. As a result, HPAI strains of the influenza virus keep epidemiologists and virologists up at night, thinking about the possibility of a future killer "bird flu" pandemic.

I want to pause here, near the beginning of our journey into the world of virologists and epidemiologists throughout the 2009 H1N1 pandemic, in order to stress the intricate web of relations—both biological and social—between viruses and humans. It is not just that we study viruses such as influenza, work with them to produce knowledge and vaccines, or that we become ill as a result of coming into contact with them, but that we *live* with them and thus, in many ways, have become viral ourselves. But that is only part of the story, since humans have arguably always been viral. Further research into junk DNA in the human genome (which, ironically, accounts for a far larger portion of the genome than segments of DNA that actively code for genes) suggests that not only is junk DNA mostly composed of remnants of viruses, but that such viral "junk" may be responsible for our own evolution and ability to fight off infection. At first, such noncoding regions of the human genome were considered simply "parasitic," remnants of old genes no longer in use (Dawkins 1976). Now scientists think that "jumping genes" or transposons in the human genome—hot spots of genetic mutation—might be responsible for the creation of new genes and for the immune system's ability to adapt to new infections.[5] If scientist-scholars like Richard Dawkins and Lynn Margulis are correct, and the latest genetic research would seem to imply that they are, then all complex organisms can be considered the result of prior symbiotic parasitic mergers between simpler organisms. In essence, then, humans are really just advanced viruses with smart phones and shoes. Our uniqueness is due to viruses' unique biological capacity to evolve.

But biologically unique or no, our distant cousins or not, viruses—let's face it—remain largely misunderstood. We instinctively recoil just at the thought of them, as though thinking of viral strains too long might make us more vulnerable to them. By spraying our countertops, squirting antimicrobial solution on our hands, washing everything with bleach, and taking antivirals we try to eradicate them and wring our collective hands when—despite our best efforts—they advance. But influenza viruses aren't really good or bad things in and of themselves; viruses are strands of RNA. Viruses don't have motives, or thoughts, or diabolical plans to wreak havoc in our cities. Their function and purpose (if we can even say that they have one) is to replicate, to evolve, to survive. They exist, in fact, because they exist. And that, I think, is what scares us the most. But if we managed to get past all the fear, panic, and disgust that viruses generate in us, what might we be able to learn about ourselves from them, about what it means to be human? The resultant "anthropology of the viral" or *viral anthropology* might allow us to explore similarities in the fundamental properties of human culture and viral cultures.

Toward a Viral Anthropology

Viral anthropology—or doing an anthropology of the viral—is not necessarily about viruses. Rather, it centers on what the terms "virus" and "viral" are used to indicate or signify in the twenty-first century: an object of study; a means of transmission; promiscuities of multiple contacts between persons, places, and things; adaptability and its relationship to evolution and survival; the vulnerability of systems and the paradox of simplicity and fragility as a type of resilience against chaos; the relationship between living and nonliving things. The possibilities, as it were, are as endless as the genetic combinations of our viral cousins.

I began thinking about viral anthropology as part of the Emergent Networks, Distributed Sensemaking (ENDS) project at Berkeley. A collaboration between epidemiology, public health, and political science, ENDS was an interdisciplinary attempt to examine and analyze how information flows through global health networks. The primary investigators (PIs) on the project were interested in how individuals, groups, agencies, and institutions coped with uncertainty. In essence, they wanted to study how people made sense of a situation or event as it developed, what types of information were crucial to the process of collective decision-making, and how people communicated across agency boundaries and international borders. It was an ambitious set of tasks, and what first struck me about working on the project was how honest the PIs were about the challenges involved in conducting such a large-scale investigation. With multiple field sites in the United States, Europe, and Asia, the sheer logistics of doing commensurate research seemed daunting enough. Adding to the project's complexity was the fact that no study quite as large or as interdisciplinary had ever been attempted. We were in uncharted research waters and while we all had universal goals in common, no one seemed entirely certain what type of methodology would work best to accomplish them. In the end, field researchers were given only a set of research questions; our individual methodologies would be dependent upon our respective fields and our own judgment.

From the start, then, communication and understanding—not only between subjects of our study but as mirrored in our own scholarly attempts to craft an interdisciplinary study—were complex and pernicious problems. Each of the field researchers kept a daily log of their activities and conversations. Posted each night on a secure web server, the logs gave us access to one another's experiences and insights. As I read over the daily field reports of my fellow researchers, I began to wonder what the collective end product of our group research might be. All of us also began to worry about fragmentation and the very ability of such a diverse assemblage of people to generate anything of broad interest. Collectively, we were trying to sort out just what this thing we were studying *was*: The "global public health network," or simply "global public health," or just particular "national and local health agencies"? Was the network of experts emergent or evolving? Were we studying one network or event—the 2009 H1N1 outbreak response—or the many day-to-day events of a complex system in action? Was everything dependent upon the particular disease or outbreak, or could we generalize what we were experiencing in an influenza pandemic to say something about the routine operations of surveillance and response in "global public health"? These were not small questions.

Sometimes it seemed as though all we had were questions and there would never be definitive answers. And yet, patterns began to emerge. We began to sense that what we were experiencing was a moment in history as it unfolded. More than that, however, as researchers in the field we began to suspect that we were all becoming a part of a superorganism, and that what we were really studying were smaller networks that linked up to form ever larger networks that together formed the entity known as global public health.

In a very real way, we were all mimicking the viruses we were trying to understand, to study, or to control. We were studying the human cultures that researched virus cultures, composed of networks of viral expertise. And as a human being that happened to be a medical anthropologist, I became very much aware that our own processes and practices as social scientists, virologists, and epidemiologists—especially in terms of information-sharing—were uncannily virus-like. In the field, I often traded information with informants; global public health operated, as it were, as a gift economy. One had to have a dowry of useful information in order to be trusted, in order to gain access to other pieces of valuable information. One scientist summed up the value of these daily information exchanges succinctly: "If you show up at my door with nothing, then you will get nothing. But if you have information to share, then it will help to create our relationship." Once I became practiced at this lateral swapping of information, I realized that as researchers we were individual virus-like nodes in an ever-emergent network of expertise. We mixed and mingled within our scientific and epidemiological "host cells," exchanging bits of partial information and reassorting it back into new configurations—like viruses swapping gene segments—all in order to understand something larger about expertise, decision making, and how we know what we know about something like a pandemic. The result was a network of viral expertise.

Indeed, we live in a viral culture. By this I mean that we live inside cultures that are constantly evolving; human cultures are all about replication, transmission, and mutation. Individuals in this viral culture are necessarily involved in a continual process of adaptation. *Information is everything in a viral culture*—it is the medium in which we work, breathe, play, die, create, and think. A viral network, in my conceptualization of it, is any group of individuals, institution, technologies, and other living and non-living things that are interconnected in an exponentially expanding web of knowledge and information-sharing. Viral anthropology is the study of those networks. It attends to the practices, thoughts, actions, kinship, and beliefs that make up the ever-transforming viral cultures of the twenty-first century. It considers the virus as a productive trope for understanding "life" as we know it.

Viral anthropology's method here is pathography; its object of study is amorphous, fuzzy, and continually evolving events and information about those events, and its field is not only multisited but constantly in motion. Viral anthropology requires a new vigilance to the ways in which humans and things interact to produce cultures. It considers the questions of information, technology, and what it means to be human in the digital age to be its defining problems. In order to do this, viral anthropology does not shy away from the anthropomorphization—or *viro*morphization[6]—of objects or institutions. Indeed, taking "things" like global public health seriously as organisms capable of a certain type of agency is a necessary part of its project.

Thus, if I anthropomorphize influenza viruses in this pathography, I also humanize other nonbiological things, too, like the CDC or the city of Hong Kong, in order to make sense out of the events of 2009 and 2010. And why not? Institutions and cities have their roles to play here. To tell a true pathography, one must at least try to let the key informants "speak" for themselves; I have chosen to make the influenza virus and global public health itself my two main protagonists. In relationship to networks and cultures, I argue that we are, in essence, already "networked in" with viruses. It is this conception of a larger, quasi-*sentient*, viral network that drew me back to a reexamination—and eventual exhumation—of the much older idea of the superorganism.[7] My argument throughout this book is that what happened during the 2009–10 H1N1 influenza pandemic can only begin to be grasped through an examination of multiple layers of experience. In order to accomplish this task effectively, I temporarily suspend here any ingrained disbelief that an institution or network of actors such as the CDC can be anthropomorphized and talked about as an organism. In what follows, therefore, I examine not only how people come to understand what "flu" is, but how the CDC, the WHO, or "global health" as a *superorganism* comprehends—or remembers and partially forgets—influenza pandemics.

On Organization

Pandemics have no real organization, beginning, or end. For this reason, there is no innate linearity to this pathography of the 2009 H1N1 pandemic. In essence, then, I have chosen an artificial device that has very real analytical uses. The organization of this book mimics the genetic organization of a virus. This pathography consists of seven chapters that are labeled as viral gene segments (with the epilogue acting as the eighth—and final—segment). Together, they form an outline of and explore the network of viral expertise that operated throughout the 2009 H1N1 influenza pandemic. Each chapter is connected to the next functionally and yet, individually, each segment tells us something different about the pandemic-at-large and about the day-to-day workings of the superorganism that is global public health. Readers may partially reconstruct their own viral anthropology of the 2009 pandemic, then, by reassorting the following chapters/gene segments at will.

Chapter 1 (segment PB2) and chapter 2 (segment PB1), examine various aspects of the science of Influenza A viruses. Chapter 1 discusses the practice of evolutionary virology and early attempts to genetically sequence the H1N1 virus during the 2009 pandemic. In this chapter, both the virus and its phylogenic tree become dual protagonists in a story about the interpretation of scientific data and the production of networks of viral expertise. Chapter 2 then explores inside a microbiology lab that looks for and sequences viral RNA from soil samples collected throughout Hong Kong and Guangdong. Here I highlight the everyday routines and practices of dealing with viral material in a "typical" lab and highlight how scientists are trained to work with individual viruses to produce knowledge about a class of viruses. These chapters work together and operate at a micro level in order to analyze the "biological" and "social" narratives of the 2009 pandemic, but also examine the practices that construct and undergird scientific knowledge and expertise about flu writ large.

Chapter 3 (segment PA) extends and shifts the examination of scientific practices and knowledge production by focusing on different—but intimately related—aspects of Hong Kong's experience with "having the flu." Here our pathography shifts from biological and social to political and cultural narratives and back again. This chapter begins by analyzing Hong Kong's "postcolonial temporality"—a term I deploy in order to capture the city's geographic and cultural positioning as being somewhere between China and "the West," and between the postcolonial past and a global future. Examining Hong Kong's century-long history as both a source of contagion and a resource for infectious disease research, this chapter ultimately explores how local epidemiologists and government officials understand and explain the decision to quarantine during the 2009 H1N1 pandemic in relationship to their epidemiological past and unique position in the superorganism of global public health. Geography, history, and culture matter not only to the interpretation and evaluation of epidemiological data during a pandemic, but to the construction of epidemiological knowledge writ large.

Chapters 4 (segment HA) and 5 (segment NP) shift our pathography from the micro to the macro level by taking a critical look at the larger history of "the flu" as an object of international concern, research, and preparedness. Past and present narratives concerning the "next big pandemic"—especially those related to the ubiquitous threat of avian influenza or H5N1—have shaped the ways in which both scientific experts and the "laity" think about the flu. Chapter 4 examines how the specter of a future deadly global pandemic of avian influenza spurred a fascination in global health policy reminiscent of the mythical danger of listening to the Greek Sirens' song. The Sirens, in this case the influenza viruses themselves, promise to reveal an ultimate knowledge of the future—an enticement few of us would have the ability to resist. Chapter 5 breaks away from scientific and historical narratives to deal with a macro level of analysis, or the political and cultural ramifications of influenza pandemics. It examines the seemingly new paradigm shift within global public health from a scientific "certainty" to a biological and situational "uncertainty" as one of the foundations of response to infectious disease outbreaks.

Chapter 6 (segment NA) focuses on the entwining of individual and collective knowledge and experience that impacts how experts come to understand and respond to something like a global pandemic. This chapter of the pathography is a viral anthropology of the production, collection, and sharing of epidemiological information during a pandemic. Scientific facts about the virus, outbreaks, and clinical cases freely circulated, but their cultural and political interpretations needed to be continuously negotiated. Expertise and context played an enormous role in how epidemiologists determined which information counted as "good" information throughout the "data deluge" that was the 2009 H1N1 pandemic. Hence, this chapter explores how experts utilize and combine historical, biological, social, individual, political, economic, and cultural narratives in order to produce "actionable knowledge" during a pandemic.

Chapter 7 (segment M1/M2) moves back to the individual and micro level to examine the personal stories of two "heretic" scientists in microbiology. Both heretics and orthodox have spent a lifetime working on viruses, and their combined narratives as laboratory scientists and epidemiologists not only reflect the state of their fields today, but reveal their own personal insights into the nature of our all too human conception of the microbial world that viruses and bacteria inhabit. In sum, heretics call for a new epistemology that conceptualizes microbes not as enemies but as co-inhabitors of our worlds and, in this way, challenge the reigning influenza research paradigm. Should the adventurous reader choose to begin this book with the last chapter first, it might alter the ways in which the rest of the gene segments are pieced together. In many ways, this final chapter highlights the "culture" of global public health through the competing personal narratives of those working inside or at the edges of it.

In the epilogue, or gene segment NS1/NS2, I reflect on my own personal journey as an anthropologist of viruses and global public health and hint at frameworks for further research in a viral anthropology of disease and global public health and a nascent anthropology of information. I argue that the messiness of events such as pandemics requires a different lens to analyze them well. In other words, a pathography can never end neatly.

1

SEEING THE PAST OR TELLING THE FUTURE?

On the Origins of Pandemics and the Phylogeny of Viral Expertise

> It is so difficult to find the beginning. Or, better: it is difficult to begin at the beginning. And not try to go further back.
>
> LUDWIG WITTGENSTEIN, *On Certainty*

Gene Segment PB2. Biological function: *Encodes a protein that slices open a host cell's mRNA (messenger RNA), producing a short primer used to begin the process of viral transcription. In human influenza viruses, PB2 also interacts with the host cell's mitochondria, inhibiting the cell's natural immune response. The biological pathway for this second function is unknown.* Pathographic function: *Examines a key biological or scientific narrative about the origins of influenza pandemics. This segment slices opens our pathography of the 2009 H1N1 pandemic by first defining its protagonist—the H1N1 virus itself—and depicting how a "pandemic" becomes a pandemic in the first place. An exploration of the production of genetic phylogenies, this segment is the primer that begins our exploration of viral expertise and the production of knowledge during the 2009 pandemic. Knowledge about a virus's genetic lineage is interpreted and used differently by virologists and epidemiology to carry out different tasks.*

On Origins

In late March 2009, a new strain of the Influenza A (H1N1) virus began to unfurl out of a remote region in Mexico. It seemed to many as if the developing pandemic might be the denouement of a harrowing story that public health workers had been telling and retelling for decades. Epidemiologists and virologists working on viruses have been sounding warning sirens about the potential for another lethal—and global—outbreak of infectious disease since the discovery of HIV/AIDS in the early eighties. Sporadic admonitions related to the collective weakness of our pandemic preparedness highlighted the very real threat posed by such emergent or "novel" viruses. These forewarnings only intensified after the 2003 SARS epidemic and in the wake of increasingly frequent outbreaks of "bird flu" in East Asia beginning in 1997. For a brief moment in the spring of 2009, then, it appeared as if all the past predictions about the epidemic future were finally coming to pass.

But were they?

And perhaps more importantly, how would we know?

Answering this all too urgent question would ultimately rely upon an understanding of what a novel Influenza A virus is in the first place, where the term "novel" is used to indicate not only biological or genetic variance but also a particular viral strain's potential for causing a deadly pandemic in an immunologically naïve population.[1] But how does the public health community come to a conclusion about whether or not a virus is both novel and dangerous enough to warrant attention and formulation of an aggressive global response? How do virologists and epidemiologists tell the difference between routine changes in seasonal influenza and modifications that could presage a killer pandemic?

Such questions are never easy to answer, but they pose a particularly thorny set of problems during a potential crisis situation as it is developing, when the speed and accuracy of decision-making matter more than ever. Throughout my fieldwork during the 2009 H1N1 pandemic, I discovered that the answers revolved almost entirely around a complex set of relationships and exchanges among evolutionary virologists, epidemiologists, and the influenza viruses that they study. As a social scientist caught up in the puzzle of determining the severity of the 2009 Influenza A (H1N1) virus, I found all the myriad social and professional exchanges vexing to trace.

Mapping out the connections between people and places necessitated an almost continuous rethinking of how we experience and embody our social and professional connections through time in an increasingly digital age. The experts I encountered thought about themselves and their work in association not only with other people, places, and institutions, but also in terms of a complicated and mutating relationship to the past and the future.

By late summer 2010, as I began to write the pathography of the pandemic, I realized I was entangled in my own temporal dilemma. The WHO had officially declared the global pandemic over, and yet I discovered that I still had far less perspective on events than any thoughtful scholar attempting to write a "factually accurate" account might desire or require of herself. I chose—perhaps artificially—to begin my initial examination of the 2009 H1N1 pandemic through an analysis of the biology of the virus. Biology and genetics might seem a peculiar place to begin any investigation of the historical origins of a particular virus or pandemic, but it becomes far more appropriate to the task at hand once one considers how the spread of a particular strain of influenza virus becomes labeled as a "pandemic" in the first place. In retrospect, beginning within the realm of the scientific laboratory also seemed like a good choice primarily because examining the biology of the virus, explaining H1N1 through its virology and genetic makeup, would be "easier" than examining its social, political, and economic aspects. It would delineate what I meant when I referred to H1N1; in effect, it would ground my pathography by defining my protagonist (and public health's antagonist)—the object at the very center of the 2009 pandemic.

Once I began the painstaking process of reviewing scientific articles, re-interviewing virologists and epidemiologists, and going through my copious field notes, however, I realized almost immediately that I had been horrifically naïve in my initial assumptions. The biological beginnings of the 2009 A (H1N1) influenza virus are anything but simple. In fact, the biological—or scientific—story is one of the trickiest narratives about the H1N1 virus, or the resulting pandemic, to recount or analyze. It is, if you will, an always mutating or drifting narrative. As any virologist can tell you, viruses are forever in flux.

Any attempt to retell the tale of the 2009 pandemic, whether beginning from the history of influenza pandemics, or from the threat of avian influenza, or from global funding for international influenza surveillance networks, or from the social and political aspects of decision-making during a pandemic, eventually leads back to biology—to the genetic sequence of the virus—and converges upon the moment that the virus first became "known" or understandable. A virus's unique genetic sequence is often conceptualized as a kind of scientific Rosetta Stone, essential not only for an accurate reading of a virus's present (or sudden presence on the global stage), but for working out its evolutionary past and predicting its epidemic future. From an evolutionary virology standpoint, the genetic sequence of an influenza virus is integral to answering the central question: *Where did this virus come from and how does it work?* And yet, as any evolutionary virologist will tell you, the predictive qualities of phylogenetic trees (or the evolutionary "lineage" charts of viruses) are deficient. Still, from the standpoint of epidemiology or public health, the genetic sequence provides crucial information about a virus's virulence, its severity, its transmissibility. For epidemiologists, genetic phylogeny is seen as "good enough" to serve as the foundation for scientific "best guesses" regarding a novel influenza virus's pandemic potential.

In this chapter, I am interested in how phylogenic trees of the H1N1 virus became central to the enactment of virological expertise as well as to the decision-making process of epidemiologists during the 2009 pandemic. From an anthropological perspective, then, genetic phylogeny is key to understanding how the social comes to insert itself into the biological and back again, or how human culture invades viral cultures and vice versa. The story of a pandemic or a particular influenza virus cannot simply be told from the singular perspective of science, or history, or epidemiology, or culture. A virus's genetic lineage is much more complicated than that; it refuses any simple explanation of its being in the world, just as it defies any traditional methods of taxonomy. Here I utilize the sequencing of influenza viruses and their resulting genetic phylogeny trees—or evolutionary trees—as an anthropological lens. In what follows, I trace the ways in which speculation about a future deadly influenza pandemic shaped not only the direction of scientific research on influenza viruses, but also helped to formulate the possible ways in which virologists and epidemiologists conceptualized the pandemic in March 2009. Our historical "pandemic past" was used not only to anticipate the epidemiological future or to influence action in the present, but helped to create the network of experts working on influenza. I take seriously the ways in which the various experts I interacted with were "tacking back and forth between the past, present and future" (Adams, Murphy, and Clarke 2009, 255) in their attempts to make better decisions about which actions to take in March 2009, a moment when it was still highly uncertain whether or not the H1N1 virus would develop into a deadly influenza pandemic. The routine practice of genetically mapping influenza viruses not only highlights biological connections among viruses through time and space, but also produces and reifies larger social structures. Genetic information is exchanged rapidly and widely among participants in the scientific network. The resultant network of information collected, analyzed, and shared is both representative and generative of the superorganism that is global public health. The playful idea of a resultant "phylogeny" of viral expertise is my attempt to highlight all the complex relationships that develop between scientists, farmers, public health institutions, and even the viruses themselves, or what the scientists themselves often referred to as "alliances" between "partners." In this framing, viruses and their genetic phylogeny trees are both derivative and constructive of biological and social relationships.

In the end, I suggest, the evolutionary tree of a virus is often "read" by virologists and epidemiologists as a type of kinship chart; by reading a phylogenic tree, one can arguably be said to know the origin story of a particular virus. But what stands out—especially in the process of discovering, analyzing, and naming a virus—is not the biological heritage of a particular viral strain, or its relationships to places, people and other objects—but its centrality to the "enactment of expertise" (Carr 2010), the assessment of risk, and the emergence of the global public health network. Nodes in the global public health network are fashioned through work done on the influenza virus, so it should also not be all that surprising if those same interpersonal and institutional relationships ultimately reflect certain characteristics of the phylogenic trees crafted through the process of sequencing, analyzing, and sharing genetic information. This chapter ultimately examines not only how a pandemic becomes a pandemic in the first place, but also how human cultures and viral cultures intersect to produce expertise.

A Brief History of Flu Research and Pandemic Planning

When an unusual late-season outbreak of an influenza-like illness hit central Mexico in March 2009, it is no surprise that epidemiologists who responded to the growing epidemic instantaneously thought of influenza. In many ways, since pandemic planning efforts began in 2003, epidemiologists had never stopped thinking of it. Public health experts were primed to respond to the beginnings of a new influenza pandemic. After the 2009 virus was subtyped as a descendant of the infamous 1918 H1N1 strain, influenza experts immediately began to worry that it might be the start of "the next big one" for which they had all been preparing. Hence there is no way to talk about the 2009 H1N1 pandemic without recourse to both the 1918 H1N1 pandemic and the more recent predictions of a potential H5N1 pandemic. This is a pathography of the 2009 pandemic, but it is also—of necessity—a story about the interrelationship between the past and future that often drives decision-making in the present moment.

Whenever I asked about the history of scientific research on influenza, when it began or how Influenza A came to be at the center of a global surveillance program, virologists or epidemiologists had to pause to think. Despite a renewed sense of urgency, which began after 9/11 in the wake of the anthrax attacks that same fall, research on potentially hazardous microbes such as influenza had already been ongoing for decades. For the "flu people," sometimes also referred to as "flu guys" since the majority of people who specialize in influenza are male, flu research already seemed ubiquitous. It is their natural milieu, and hence it is hard for them to put an exact date on its beginnings. The history of influenza itself is no less elusive. Medical historians have identified outbreaks of an influenza-like disease in historical records dating as far back as Greece in 412 BC. The first medical description of an outbreak of influenza was recorded in Philadelphia as early as 1793 (Oldstone 1998, 179). But the events which form the backbone of this pathography span the more recent history of the field of influenza virology.

It is not at all spurious to argue that everything began in 1918. A pandemic of H1N1 Influenza A virus that year impelled what has now become almost a century's worth of intense scientific study on a single infectious disease agent. During the deadly 1918 pandemic, which lasted approximately eighteen months, it is estimated that between twenty and forty million people died worldwide as a result of the flu. As millions of people fell ill and died in record numbers, an animal husbandry inspector working for the US government noticed that swine on farms were falling prey to a disease with a similar set of symptoms. Over a decade of subsequent research on porcine influenza provided scientists with concrete evidence that influenza is caused by a virus (and not a bacterium, as had been suspected). Even so, the influenza virus was not isolated and confirmed in a laboratory using Koch's postulates[2] until 1932 (Potter 2001), during a relatively minor epidemic of influenza subsequent to the 1918 pandemic. During that epidemic, researchers at Wellcome Laboratories in London who became infected with influenza noticed that ferrets in their research facility also fell ill,[3] and quickly confirmed that influenza was transmitted via virus (Oldstone 1998, 181). In essence, this single event marks the official start of modern influenza virology.

For the following two decades, laboratory research on influenza progressed slowly. In 1941, the HA and NA surface proteins were first described, and their usefulness as markers for detecting and tracking influenza viruses was immediately recognized (Artenstein 2010, 194). The discovery of the roles of these surface proteins in invading a host cell also helped to advance the biological understanding of how influenza functioned. At the same time, beginning in 1940 and continuing throughout the 1950s, MacFarlane Burnet, an Australian scientist, made significant progress in the use of chicken embryos for research on influenza. He established the practice of cultivating influenza viruses in eggs (Oldstone 1998, 182)—a technological advance that made it possible not only to grow large amounts of the virus for scientific study and diagnostic assays, but also enabled the development of influenza vaccines.[4]

Given that World War I had precipitated the deadliest influenza pandemic in memory, the United States had influenza near the top of its list of concerns as it approached World War II. Preparations for that war included the establishment of a Commission on Influenza (Artenstein 2010, 198), which would be instrumental in the development of effective vaccines. World War II also inaugurated the practice of mass vaccination campaigns among US soldiers, thereby providing virologists and epidemiologists with their first chance to study vaccine effectiveness in a large population. The Commission on Influenza financed a bevy of scientific research over the three decades of its existence, and spurred broader advancements in research on other viral pathogens. By 1957, when another pandemic of influenza spread around the globe, virologists and epidemiologists were equipped with far better methods and equipment (Artenstein 2010, 200), marking the beginnings of modern virological analysis of Influenza A. Since then, laboratory work on influenza has progressed apace, increasingly reliant upon new techniques in genetic sequencing and analysis, and focused on unpacking the virus's origins, understanding its ecological environment, and decoding its biological processes and functioning inside host cells. With the establishment of the WHO's Global Influenza Surveillance Network (GISN)[5] in 1952, and the network's expansion over the ensuing decades, laboratory research on influenza continues to receive a generous amount of international attention and funding.

The history of scientific research on the influenza virus is, of course, deeply intertwined with that of pandemic planning. Did advances in virological analysis of the virus spur increased surveillance and planning efforts? Or did military and national security needs—with their attendant focus on pandemic planning and preparedness—ultimately drive scientific research on influenza? It is nearly impossible to assert that either influenza research or planning has primacy over the other; rather, the two have co-evolved in a symbiotic relationship from 1952, with the establishment of GISN, to the present day. At the time of this writing, in the spring of 2013, influenza research and planning seemed both already naturalized and unquestionably necessary. So much so that many virologists and epidemiologists had trouble articulating its long history. And yet there *is* a traceable historical trajectory—one might even label it a genealogical one—from the pandemic of 1918 to the pandemic of 2009 and beyond.

Fast-forward to 1993, the year that virologist Stephen S. Morse edits the influential book, *Emerging Viruses*. The volume reflects the collective expertise of some of the most famed and respected virologists and is a call to arms—or at least a plea for more awareness, vigilance, and increased funding for research. Morse and his colleagues argue that emerging viruses, defined as "viruses that either have newly appeared in the population or are rapidly expanding their range, with a corresponding increase in cases of disease" (10), threaten the human population as a whole. Viruses, Richard Krause, a senior scientific adviser to the NIH, reminds readers in the foreword, "know no country" (xvii) and thus require international cooperation and global surveillance and planning. Morse and his contributors argue that "viral traffic" (17), or movement of viruses from one species to another, represented perhaps the single biggest threat to health. The first "emergent" viral threat to be explored in the volume is influenza, in an essay written by renowned virologist Robert G. Webster (more on Webster and the "phylogeny" of modern influenza research and expertise below).

Webster underscores the potential lethality of influenza viruses, ending with reference to the 1918 strain, and highlighting the need for continuous surveillance of genetic shifts in the many Influenza A subtypes that make their home in wild birds.

Morse's book had a tremendous effect on public health policy and scientific funding in the following decade. In many ways, the volume represented a pivotal shift in scientific and public health policy on viruses. It also sparked a renewed public attention to viral diseases and the potential horrors of future pandemics, which reached a crescendo in 1995 with the publication of journalist Laurie Garrett's book *The Coming Plague* and the release of the Hollywood movie *Outbreak*. Then, in 1997, the first case of "bird flu" or H5N1 in a human was detected in Hong Kong. Fears of another 1918-like pandemic began to mount almost immediately; the threat of another influenza pandemic engendered not only an increased focus on virus surveillance, but a new fervor in public health planning. In 2003, a quickly spreading, international outbreak of a novel and lethal coronavirus—descriptively named Severe Acute Respiratory Syndrome (SARS)—made the need for comprehensive national pandemic plans seem even more urgent. In the aftermath of SARS, continued sporadic outbreaks of "bird flu" or H5N1—and the avian influenza virus's spread to new geographic areas—made a future influenza pandemic appear more and more certain. People in public health circles began to talk of "when," not "if," in relationship to a repeat of the 1918 pandemic. By 9/11, several popular nonfiction books about the 1918 influenza pandemic and "bird flu" were already in circulation. The World Trade Center and anthrax attacks merely aggravated an existent anxiety in governmental, scientific, and public health circles in relationship to microbes as either natural or manmade threats to public health and national security.

By 2003, the combination of echoes of the 1918 influenza pandemic, renewed attention to viruses in the wake of HIV/AIDS, the continued appearance of sporadic H5N1 Influenza A cases in Asia and Africa, the international spread of SARS, and an increased attention to biological agents as part of possible terrorist attacks had combined to foment a universal call for better public health planning and preparedness.[6] The WHO directed efforts by revising the International Health Regulations to include "operational aspects" for coordination of the international response to outbreaks of infectious disease, crafting a pandemic phase system, and issuing its Global Influenza Preparedness Plan (World Health Organisation 2005), urging all member nations to formulate their own national pandemic plans. Indeed, by 2005, "pandemic planning" had become all but synonymous with influenza preparedness. Influenza had become a paradigmatic infectious disease, the virus at the center of global surveillance, research, and planning efforts.[7]

The Quest for Origins: Taxonomy, Relatedness, and the Production of Genetic Phylogeny

Throughout my research, it seemed to me as if the answer to almost every question regarding the 2009 H1N1 influenza pandemic spiraled out from a strand of its viral RNA. At times, the tendrils of genetic material seemed to be stretching themselves out like a webby net, catching all of us up in the collective thrill of deciphering a pandemic's future by reading about its viral past. I was as guilty as any epidemiologist of hoping that a random series of nucleotides might provide answers to all our collective questions about the developing pandemic.

When virologists talk about a "novel" or reemergent strain of virus, they often directly refer to the virus's genealogy. In a lab I visited in Hong Kong, a genealogical tree of H5N1 masked the entire backside of the PI's office door. Particular segments had been highlighted in yellow and handwritten notes covered the broad margins. Printouts showing other viral linkages were carefully taped together and completely covered the otherwise empty wall spaces next to work desks throughout the lab. Examples of these phylogeny trees were everywhere—the visible product of the material processes of virus discovery and genetic sequencing. The printouts were used variously for reference and for discussion, but they were also signals of expertise hung on the walls like diplomas or certificates. They were indications of the production of knowledge as much as they grounded the continuous search for new genetic information from viral samples.

Genetic phylogeny is the scientific term used to refer to a virus's particular evolutionary history, but many of the actual terms and phrases utilized by scientists mapping out the genealogy of a virus mirror the more familiar social expressions used to describe familial relationships between persons or groups of persons. A virus is frequently described as a member of or related to a "family" of viruses, or as simply a "descendant" of other known viruses. A virus may have close or distant "relatives," and different viruses may be said to share a "common ancestor." In leading scientific journals such as *Science* and *Nature*, the 2009 H1N1 virus was often also personified and given human-like agency and traits. One early account of the virus's biological origins went so far as to suggest that H1N1 was part of a particularly "promiscuous family" (Cohen 2009a).

Viral taxonomy, or the classification of viruses, has always been a contentious issue among scientific researchers (Matthews 1985), in part due to viruses' ability to exchange entire genetic segments with other viruses co-infecting the same cell (antigenic shift). In addition to these significant genetic changes, a virus's genetic makeup is continually changing in more subtle ways as a consequence of frequent copying mistakes during the process of replication inside a host cell (antigenic drift). The class of viruses known as Influenza A has a total of eight different gene segments, which regularly undergo both drift and shift to produce new subtypes of Influenza A viruses.

As a result of this biological complexity, the procedure for establishing scientific names for Influenza A viruses is anything but simple. According to FluGenome, a website dedicated to the development of better web tools to aid researchers in studying the evolutionary phylogeny of Influenza A viruses, the standard nomenclature should be as follows:

Two nomenclature conventions are used routinely in influenza research: 1) the 8 segments in the influenza A genome are numbered from 1 to 8 for PB2, PB1, PA, HA, NP, NA, M, and NS respectively; 2) There are currently 16 subtypes for hemagglutinin (HA), 9 subtypes for neuraminidase (NA), and 2 alleles for nonstructural (NS) proteins. Since influenza A viruses have a complicated genomic structure, we approached genotyping by studying each gene segment separately at first. According to the conventions and the fact that the evolution rate varies from segment to segment, we define a genotype as a sequential combination of the lineages for each of the eight segments in a genome, where a letter is assigned to each lineage of PB2, PB1, PA, NP, and M, and a number with a letter is assigned to each lineage of HA, NA, and NS with the number representing the subtype or allele. For example, [A, B, C, 5A, A, 1A, A, 2C] is the genotype of an H5N1 virus with the lineage A for the PB2 segment, B for PB1, C for PA, 5A for HA, and so on (the first gene listed being gene 1, the second being gene 2, and so on).

The use of a nomenclature for influenza A virus genotypes is important, since it will allow researchers to describe influenza A virus genotypes in an equivocal way and avoid the confusion when a genotype is labeled differently by researchers. (2010)

This statement reveals, implicit in its call for a more uniform nomenclature, some of the inherent problems with standardization and prior attempts to produce more interlab "clarity." In day-to-day practice, the system for naming—or labeling—unique viral segments is anything but uniform.

A particular virology lab might craft and utilize its own nomenclature system, making difficult any quick comparison of viral sequences and other information-sharing between collaborators at different institutions. Under the current system, each virology laboratory producing information on individual gene sequences might produce virus labels or nomenclature that "reads" slightly differently, making fast "translation" among labs working on the same class of viruses that much more difficult. In the lab I observed, influenza viruses were named using the following standardized system: year/month/species/identification code for host species/identification code for the specific virus sample/specific hemagglutinin and neuraminidase subtypes. When I asked the head scientist if he could easily tell me where—in geographic terms—a gene segment had originated, he responded that they were trying to formulate a way to include the known sample source location in the current nomenclature system.

In practice, however, a commonly circulating influenza virus (in distinction from a virus that is being researched on a continual basis or under "normal surveillance" in a virology lab) is often given a more generic name that reflects its approximate place of origin, its primary animal host, or its specific subtype. Thus, the 2009 A (H1N1) virus was often referred to both in the press and by professionals interchangeably as "Mexican flu," "swine flu," and "H1N1."[8] Controversies over these early nonscientific names were rife and well reported in the news media (Bradsher 2009, Grady 2009, Weeks 2009). Government officials in places like Mexico or China quickly balked at the suggestion that the flu had originated inside their national borders (McNeil 2009, China Daily 2009a, China Daily 2009b); a reaction partially explained by economic fears of halted tourism and trade, and partly by the stigma of being labeled as the "origin" of a pandemic strain of flu. The pork industry lobbied for the use of "H1N1" due to its concern that the name "swine flu" would negatively affect sales (a fear not completely unfounded considering the past effects of FMD or "Mad Cow" disease on international beef sales).[9] Nomenclature would only become a nonissue after the virus's RNA had been carefully "read" and its origins were better understood.

The various people I had conversations with during the early weeks of the pandemic—from officials of California's regional public health departments and national public health agencies to employees in supermarkets and coffee shops—all wanted to know more about this strain of flu, about where the virus had originated, where it would travel, and how it would act when it got there. What is more, many professional epidemiologists agreed that a definitive scientific answer to the puzzle of the virus's origins—or genetic phylogeny—might provide them with other vital information or insights about where the virus—and the pandemic—was headed, what shape it would take, and what public health responses would be needed in order to halt its spread.[10] In fact, people seemed to want the virus's RNA to "speak" to them, to relate its history, and to give up its secrets. Throughout 2009, I often heard discussions or perused news stories and scientific articles related to the virus's biological heritage, or its kinship to other viruses, in terms of both the distant past[11] as well as of the present and future.

It seemed particularly important to ascertain the virus's genetic sequence during the earliest days of the developing pandemic. As soon as sputum and blood samples from the first index patients (the initial cases) in California and Mexico became available, scientists began to isolate and then sequence the virus.[12] In the United States, the first samples were sent to the CDC from the Naval Medical Center in San Diego on April 13 (MMWR Weekly 2009). On April 15, the CDC used polymerase chain reaction (PCR) on the samples and confirmed that the viral strain was different from anything circulating at that time in the United States during the normal flu season (personal notes from the ENDS workshop at Berkeley, July 2009). Scientists working on samples in laboratories in Canada, the UK, and the United States made genetic sequences available on public databases. Two weeks later, on April 30, initial genetic analyses of the circulating strain were already available on a "wiki-style Web site called 'Human/Swine A/H1N1 Influenza Origins and Evolution' created by two evolutionary biologists in the United Kingdom" (Cohen 2009a, 870).

In the history of public health flu surveillance and response, the rapidity of the sequencing and evolutionary analysis of the 2009 A (H1N1) virus was unprecedented.

So much so that epidemiologists and scientists working within public health were stunned, and continually expressed admiration for the collaborative international efforts that had produced such useful information, under strain and demanding time constraints to boot. A prominent French epidemiologist recalled his own reaction a few months later, stating that "The genetic sequence was published very, very quickly. I remember seeing it in the *New England Journal of Medicine* and thinking to myself, 'Wow. This is terrific, to have this kind of information so quickly.' And it seemed like it was done properly. It was good science" (personal notes from the ENDS workshop at Berkeley, July 2009). While working inside the CDC during the fall of 2009, I continually heard people working on the H1N1 response remark on how quickly information had become available in the early days of the outbreak, how easily information had been shared between global partners,[13] and how smoothly the scientific community had churned out not only the complete genetic sequence of the virus, but comparative data regarding its evolutionary origins. The partial "origin story" constructed through the available circulating data on the virus's genetic structure was, then, an artifact of these very technological collaborations. The genetic sequence of this novel virus was thus the successful product not just of the individual actors, but of the superorganism that was the network of world experts on influenza.

In many ways the speed and style of collaboration that produced expert knowledge about the genetic makeup of the 2009 H1N1 virus mirrored the ability of Influenza A viruses to readily swap information. In point of fact, the sequence analysis of the virus was available long before the outbreak had even officially been declared a pandemic by the WHO. Epidemiologists reacted to this as if a small miracle had occurred. Long after the sequence was published, the professionals I interviewed both in the United States and in Hong Kong articulated something akin to wonder and delight, and often pointed to the achievement as the fait accompli of a new, better, more prepared system of global public health. A decade of pandemic planning, relationship-building exercises and workshops, and the development of sophisticated IT programs had helped to create more efficient information-sharing channels (both at the official—or governmental—levels and at the individual—or interpersonal—level). Official information-sharing websites and systems provided quick and easy access to key pieces of scientific information during the earliest days and weeks of the pandemic (see chapter 6 for a more detailed analysis of information-sharing in Global Public Health). Articles and interviews in the two leading scientific journals *Science* and *Nature* reflected this sentiment, with prominent virologists and epidemiologists declaring their "amazement" at the sequence-sharing capacity of the network (Cohen 2009b, 701), or at how quickly "people mobilized" (Cohen 2009a, 870) within it. In many ways, the sequencing of the novel H1N1 virus was seen as the first victory in the battle against the pandemic and a major blow in the larger war against "flu."

Scientists ascertained from the available genetic sequences that the circulating H1N1 pandemic virus was something called a "triple reassortant." In the lingua franca of virology, this—in essence—means that the virus is a rare combination of gene segments from viruses from three different hosts: avian, human, and swine. The 2009 A (H1N1) influenza virus, from both a scientific and quasi-anthropological standpoint, has a rather complicated genealogy; it is the unique descendant of viruses from North American pigs, North American birds, Eurasian pigs, and humans (Cohen 2009a). Still, knowing which gene segments came from which mammalian hosts or regions of the globe would not definitively answer the ultimate question that epidemiologists found themselves repeating: Where—*exactly*—had this virus come from? The answer to this question was important not only for accurately naming the virus (as explained above, a virus's origin is typically included as a part of its scientific nomenclature), but for understanding more about its initial emergence as well as its early spread and future development.

The first scientific articles on the "origins" of H1N1 read much like stories about viruses begetting viruses, on biblical lines. Biology here (and perhaps more often than we recognize) equates to the search for a beginning. To understand the virus, scientists and epidemiologists wanted to not only trace out its viral kinship chart, or to find its parents, but to reconstruct the moment of its "birth." An evolutionary virologist explained to me that while it remained scientifically impossible to ascertain exactly when, where, and how a novel virus had reassorted into its present form, the production and analysis of its genetic phylogeny could help scientists to *approximate* the origins of a particular viral strain. In essence, understanding the genetic phylogeny of H1N1 was "good enough" to explain its past, but remained a poor predictor of its ultimate future. Exactly like a newborn baby, knowing H1N1's "parents" would be little help in guessing what the "child" would become or might do as an "adult." But for many epidemiologists and public health officials, this was exactly what the search for origins was about—the ability to intervene, based on a knowledge of the past, in a virus's future. For an evolutionary virologist, the practice of producing phylogeny charts was an attempt to understand something more about a class of viruses and how they functioned *in the long term*; for the epidemiologist, reading a phylogeny chart for the H1N1 was about being able to make better decisions about pandemic response *in the short term*. It became clear that the "origins" that both groups discussed and debated were not the same object in time.

Phylogenetic trees are, in essence, important scientific objects that have slightly different uses and meanings for different groups of experts. Phylogenetic trees for viruses look similar in form to human genealogical trees, with the obvious exception being that phylogenetic trees are based on a virus's RNA structure and are thus much bigger and more intricate in terms of both scale and scope.

Still, the similarity in basic format makes the phylogenetic tree seem almost intuitively easy to understand, even from a novice's perspective. Phylogeny trees are produced for each of the eight separate segments of an influenza virus (which viewed together constitute the entire genetic evolutionary tree for the virus as a whole). Typically, however, emphasis is placed on the specific gene segments that encode hemagglutinin (HA) and neuraminidase (NA), two proteins that cover the outer surface of an influenza virus and are crucial to its ability to invade a host cell and effectively replicate. Both HA and NA also have a "very high" rate of mutation, due largely to continual selection pressure from the immune systems of their mammalian hosts (Webster et al. 1992, 155). Information gathered through continual surveillance[14] and sequencing of Influenza A viruses is used to track longitudinal changes in an effort to better understand how viruses mutate and reassort into "novel"—and potentially deadly—strains (which are typically hybrids of strains found in a variety of animal hosts: ducks, wild geese, pigs, humans, and chickens).

From an anthropological or science studies perspective, the construction of these phylogenetic trees also helps to create a "novel" strain in the

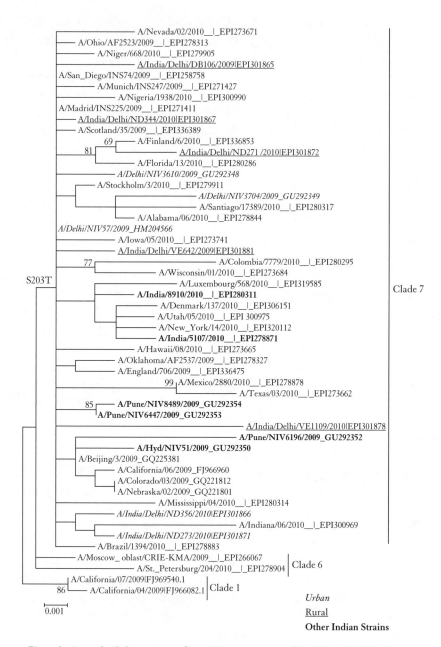

Figure 3. A sample phylogenetic tree for an HA gene segment of the 2009 A (H1N1) influenza virus collected from North India. Image from Broor et al. 2012.

first place. It is the comparison between strains through time that produces the differences that makes the difference in how we think about viral relatedness. In addition, phylogenetic *relationships between strains* are analyzed to produce knowledge about the "ecology" of influenza viruses (Webster et al. 1992). The comparison of the phylogenetic trees for individual gene segments, which began in earnest as late as the mid-1990s, led to the scientific discovery of influenza's natural host reservoirs (wild birds) and ultimately undergirds the entire scientific paradigm for evolutionary research on influenza viruses. Viral sequence data are thus absolutely essential to the work of present-day evolutionary virologists, who track and compare specific changes in nucleotide and amino acid sequences of gene segments to produce information on the known origins, or most recent common ancestor, of seasonal and pandemic flu strains.

A Brief Phylogeny of the "Flu Guys": A Network that Trains and Researches Together Develops Expertise Together

After even a cursory reading of available scientific literature, the close connection between phylogeny, scientific nomenclature, and "kinship" between viruses is unmistakable. What I am interested in here, however, is not just how the production of phylogeny trees highlights or produces biological relationships between viruses, but how the trees themselves—as virologists' attempts to accurately reflect the virus's biological makeup and history—mirror or refract a social relationality among the experts themselves. Virologists are "related" to each other, and their relationships might be mapped onto the very phylogeny trees that they produce; these "fraternal" bonds can be traced through their histories of professional training, their citational practices, and their processes of sharing virus samples, lab methods, and genetic information. Such a "phylogeny of viral expertise" would likely be as messy to construct and to interpret as the viral phylogeny trees themselves.

The heart of this surveillance and research program is a "family" of influenza viruses (Influenza A) and its attendant "family" of researchers, an interlaced network of individuals that helps to shape—both physically and semantically—the world of influenza science. At the center of the network is virologist Robert Webster. In many ways, Webster's personal history reads like the history of influenza science itself. The collection of scientific articles written or co-authored by Webster (his professional web page at St. Jude's Hospital lists this number as over 650 and counting) can in turn be analyzed to produce a "tree" or web of genealogical and material[15] relatedness among influenza researchers. Most influential evolutionary virologists working on influenza have either been trained by Webster, worked with him, or rely upon his work as foundational to their own. Over the past decade, Webster has been inducted into the Royal Society in London (the oldest scientific society in the world) and the National Academy of Sciences, acted as a consultant to the WHO and the National Institute of Allergy and Infectious Disease, and is the director of the US Collaborating Center of the WHO for the ecology of animal influenza viruses (Webster 2013). In essence, Dr. Robert Webster is a prominent and highly respected virologist and founding figure of the field of evolutionary virology of influenza. His opinion matters greatly to other practitioners and his research is the basis for the global network of researchers now working on Influenza A viruses.

Webster began his work on influenza in 1957, when he discovered that human pandemic influenza, such as the deadly 1918 H1N1 A and the 1957 pandemic strains, had descended from viruses affecting animals and birds. The "origin story" of the pivotal founding event of his future career as an evolutionary virologist is myth-like. According to a feature article on Webster published in the *Smithsonian Magazine* (Rosenwald 2006), Webster was walking "along an Australian beach in the 1960s" with his research partner, Graeme Laver. As they "strolled," they passed a dead muttonbird—a kind of seabird—about every fifteen yards. Knowing that a flu virus had recently been pinpointed as the cause of death in birds in South Africa, Webster turned to his lab partner and asked: "What if the flu killed these birds?" The two men then embarked on a research trip together, eventually swabbing the throats of hundreds of birds; eighteen of those first samples would test positive for antibodies to the human virus that had caused the 1957 influenza pandemic. Thus, Webster and his research partner brought into being a robust research program that has lasted for over fifty years.

A quick perusal of Webster's extensive list of important publications might be productively mapped to craft a "phylogenetic tree" of influenza researchers themselves, all showing Webster as their progenitor or research "ancestor." During my research in Hong Kong, I began to think of the ways in which viruses as objects at the center of an intense scientific research program had connected a variety of people, places, and institutions. After hearing Robert Webster's name mentioned in five separate interviews with virologists (sometimes just as "Bob"), it became clear that researchers were connected in patterns that were similar in form to the phylogeny trees they studied and helped to produce. This should have been less strange to me, I suppose, since I knew that Webster had collaborated on research with the men responsible for the discovery of the SARS coronavirus, Guan Yi and Malik Peiris (prominent virologists in their own right and both currently professors at the University of Hong Kong). And yet it struck me that one could not have a conversation about evolutionary virology in Hong Kong without recourse to Robert Webster or his protégé, Richard Webby (also at St. Jude's and current Director of the WHO Collaborating Center for Studies on the Ecology of Influenza in Animals and Birds).

As the foundational researcher in evolutionary virology, Robert Webster connected people—geographically, intellectually, and materially—through their common interests or training in the virology of influenza. The virus samples, as I had seen for myself, also connected people into collaborative alliances. Together, the "common ancestor" of influenza science and the viruses had created a billion-dollar global network for surveillance and laboratory research on a single class of Influenza A viruses. If that class of viruses had complicated genealogies, then so did the scientists who studied them. Indeed, the international research focus on influenza, initially begun by Webster and Laver, had constructed behemoth global networks, such as WHO's Global Influenza Surveillance Network (GISN) and its information-sharing tool, FluNet, out of a myriad of smaller, more intimate, personal alliances. The respect that Robert Webster commanded was more or less transferable to the laboratory research practices that he had begun and continued to vocally support. At the heart of all this, however, were still the viruses themselves—a family that produced a network that produced a superorganism. As twentieth-century objects of fascination, the influenza viruses had connected and were connected by human practices—both inside and outside of the lab. As one press release from EuroSurveillance stated, the sequencing of viral isolates of the 2009 A(H1N1) influenza virus "is allowing thousands of scientists to participate in the endeavor" (Trifonov et al. 2009).

But once a phylogenetic tree is constructed by this "phylogeny of expertise," the interconnected scientific researchers working on viral isolates, how is the resultant phylogenetic information then understood—or reinterpreted—both inside and outside the virology lab? If, as prominent virologists like Robert Webster have argued, phylogenetic information should not be used to predict the future of a pandemic, then how is genetic information being utilized by epidemiologists and other public health officials? Does virological expertise based on the phylogeny of viruses translate outside the lab?

Overlapping Networks of Expertise: The Interpretation of Genetic Information within Evolutionary Virology and Epidemiology

What do these genetic sequences mean to the various experts involved in "reading" and interpreting them? More importantly, what might social scientists learn about the development and management of expertise and the creation of information-sharing networks from analyzing the routine scientific practice of producing and interpreting phylogenetic trees? E. Summerson Carr reminds us that expertise is inherently interactional and ideological. It is, then, essentially social as well as the result of material practices in the lab. Expertise is something that virologists and epidemiologists *do*, not something that they naturally *have* or acquire.[16] Evolutionary virologists are specifically trained and socialized—to borrow from Carr—to learn "how to define and frame, as well as to interpret and engage objects in an expert way" (2010, 20). The objects in question here are phylogenic trees. These working objects are central to the formation of scientific expertise within the field of global public health. As Carr notes, "would-be experts must continuously work to authenticate themselves as experts as well as to authenticate the objects of their expertise" (21). I am interested here in how these trees became central to the enactment of virological expertise as well as to the decision-making process of epidemiologists during the 2009 pandemic.

Most of the epidemiologists and analysts that I spoke with told me the same thing—that certain key pieces of information about the virus were missing during the first few days and weeks of the 2009 H1N1 outbreak: its virulence, transmissibility, and origins. Knowing the specific genetic makeup of the circulating virus might allow public health experts to make more accurate, educated guesses about the spread and severity of the flu, and this, in turn, might lead to better decisions about what types of public health responses would be most effective. In addition, being able to quickly analyze viral RNA would allow scientists to keep tabs on the virus in case it mutated or evolved into a more dangerous form.

It was essential, I was repeatedly counseled whenever I asked about the importance of continued global virological surveillance of influenza viruses, to keep track of point mutations (a change in a single base amino acid) and reassortment events (the "switching out" or "swapping" of entire gene segments resulting in antigenic shift). Evolutionary virologists think of this as part of a "basic research" paradigm, one that will eventually help them to understand how influenza viruses evolve in their natural environments. It is vital to study the complex relationship between a virus's ecology and its evolution; the virologists I interviewed believe that genetic phylogeny holds a key to unlocking the secrets of how viruses function. Generating sequences and compiling computational databases of genetic sequences across time is conceptualized by the evolutionary virologists I spoke with as creating an "oil reserve," or as a process similar to sifting through sediment layers in a "diamond or gold mine"; the more information that is gathered together and compared, the better the chances of discovering something that might enrich our understanding of viruses. But if phylogenetic information seems to hold out the promise of greater knowledge, then that promise is inherently limited.

Robert Webster, quoted in *Science*, explains the popular quest for information regarding the RNA sequences of viruses: " 'There is a feeling that once you know the sequence, you know everything about a virus, and you really don't' " (Cohen and Enserink 2009a, 573). Virologists familiar with genetic phylogeny repeatedly stressed this point in conversations, and were careful to highlight the limitations of knowing the genetic makeup and evolutionary history of a virus. But if realizing that the genetic sequence alone could not tell public health professionals everything they wanted to know about the 2009 A (H1N1) virus, that fact had not stopped anyone from racing to sequence the virus or attempting to use the resulting data to help them piece together its evolutionary history. Epidemiologists in key public health institutions attempted to utilize this newly available knowledge about the genetic makeup of H1N1 to help them make calculated predictions about the virus's spread and its potential for causing widespread death. Indeed, the CDC and the WHO eventually retooled their official recommendations for local public health action based—at least in part—upon this information.

Near the end of my research, I noticed a developing divide between what the expert virologists who produced evolutionary trees thought they *should* be used to do, and what other—less specialized—public health professionals thought they *might* be used to do. Different scientific interpretations of the phylogenetic tree of the 2009 A (H1N1) influenza virus offer us a way to further examine how the routine practice of mapping and comparing phylogeny both formulates expertise and creates an esoteric network of influenza experts. How virologists and epidemiologists talked about and conceived the intricate relationships between the 2009 virus and other viruses (such as the infamous 1918 strain)[17] often mirrored the way they discussed their own roles or positions in the phylogeny of viral expertise.

Evolutionary Virologists on Sequencing, Phylogenetic Trees, and "Gene Flows"

It is important to note that the first half of my fieldwork was spent working with epidemiologists and analysts inside the CDC. I cut my public health teeth, so to speak, on a specific formulation of the role that genetic information about a virus should play in global disease surveillance or during an outbreak response. My knowledge of the science had been colored by this immersion in the daily work of top epidemiologists, in ways that I would not fully realize until my time in Hong Kong. It was fortuitous, then, that my first meeting in Hong Kong was with a prominent evolutionary virologist who had been quoted in several high-profile media and science stories on the genetic sequencing of the 2009 A (H1N1) influenza virus. His work on the phylogenetic tree of the virus, as it were, preceded him. After I sat down with Dr. Gavin Smith to discuss influenza research in Hong Kong, my understanding of the call for more effective global infectious disease surveillance programs, and international scientific efforts to track evolutionary changes in influenza viruses, as well as to monitor exactly what RNA could—and couldn't—reveal about a virus altered dramatically.

Gavin met me on an overcast day at a popular brunch spot in Central District. He was younger than most of the people I met working on influenza, yet he had already accrued over a decade of lab experience working in the "best place to study viruses." He was frank and seemed willing to talk openly about the social and cultural politics of working on influenza in the SAR. As an internationally respected virologist, Gavin was in the loop. He had worked inside top labs and alongside scientists who were already famous infectious disease specialists (including the scientists responsible for the initial discovery of the SARS coronavirus). Gavin regularly name-dropped throughout our conversation, though in an offhand way, unself-consciously. He collaborated with renowned scientists on a regular basis, he knew them well or had trained under them, and though it was still "early" in his career, he was fast becoming one of them. In other words, although the ethnographic account here focuses only upon one evolutionary virologist's point of view, Gavin's respected position in the network of expertise is unquestionable and his views are typical of those of others I met during later stages of research. His views on the uses of phylogenetic trees are thus not atypical for his position or research focus, and indeed are paradigmatic of the ways in which evolutionary virologists typically explain their research and its limitations.

Gavin and I discussed the routine sequencing of viral samples in Hong Kong over our scones, eggs benedict, and coffee. When asked if his lab sequenced every virus found through randomized sampling and surveillance, Gavin laughed and launched into an explanation of the process of sequencing based on his recent experience with swine viruses, including H1N1:

> No, there's too many. I'll give an example from the pig stuff, because that's what we've been working on a lot recently. We're doing a lot of sequencing of the pigs. So for the pig stuff, we've got about 600 viruses—this is just H1N1—that have been isolated since 1998. So we sequence the surface proteins, the HA and NA, of all. And then we do phylogenetic analysis, and then we sort of decide what to do full genome based on the phylogeny and try to sample equally from different phylogenetic routes on the HA and NA. It's not ideal, but it's *really* expensive.[18] And then we've chosen about 30 percent, 20 to 30 percent normally, depending on what the total numbers are, and do full genome sequencing.

In twelve years, then, in only one virology lab in the Hong Kong Special Administrative Region, scientists had been able to isolate approximately six hundred virus samples of a single subtype of influenza. The genetic information generated from sequencing merely one-third of these samples would then be used to compare "nucleotide and amino acid sequences" of each virus's unique RNA, particularly changes in sequences that are found within the HA and NA gene segments. Phylogenies generated by comparisons between viruses would then be utilized to assemble viruses into a "sister group relationship" to determine "a common ancestor." These trees, in turn, are a way to "represent hypotheses about evolutionary relationships among taxa." What evolutionary virologists like Gavin Smith hope to ascertain from the information represented by phylogenetic trees is "a more complete picture of virus evolution," and a greater understanding of the ecology of viruses, even if the genetic sequences and phylogenetic trees can admittedly never be used to pinpoint the specific origin or emergence of a particular viral strain (Webster et al. 1992, 164, 167, 171).

When I mentioned Robert Webster's quote in *Science* on the origins of H1N1, Gavin smiled. I asked how good the predictive quality of the sequencing is. He responded quickly:

> Oh, it's not. You've got to biologically characterize it. You can sequence something, and say it's got a mutation that confers oseltamivir [Tamiflu] resistance. If you read the papers, what they *should* say, and hopefully what we always say, is that it is *predicted* to confer oseltamivir resistance.
>
> Because you get a nucleotide, you haven't even sequenced the amino acid, and then we just convert it using the universal code into amino acid and then it's got the resistance marker. But unless you test it—that virus—directly against that drug, you cannot say. And on a simple measure, I think that's what he's saying. But a lot of the focus on information-sharing and things like that, it's all been *information* sharing, there's not been things about viruses and sharing as such. So a lot of the criticism is, oh, you've got to provide the sequences. But what are you going to do with that? I mean, you can't actually *do* anything with it. You can look into the past, but you can't look at the future.
>
> I think the real hope is a need for real-time surveillance. What we're trying to do with it from a disease-control point of view is we're looking at gene flows. If you've got gene flows between different host populations [typically between bird, pig, and human], then past experience tells you that something's going to happen.

In his follow-up, Gavin took pains to underline that if certain genetic mutations—such as those related to drug resistance and discussed above—

are present, then a virologist could and would be very confident that the virus is resistant to drugs, without necessarily having "proof" in the form of a biological assay. Such genetic information can be useful within the context of public health. However, as Gavin emphasized, most genetic mutations, specifically ones that may be related to host specificity or host adaptation (or, in layman's terms, to a virus's capacity to infect and replicate inside a host), are far less clear in terms of their biological significance. Under limited circumstances, then, genetic sequences can be used to make decisions about how to response to a pandemic threat.

Most genetic information by itself is useless without contextual information regarding how the virus will act inside a live host in real time. And what it can tell us, according to evolutionary virologists like Robert Webster and Gavin Smith, is mostly about a virus's past, not about its present or its future, and then only with the aid of a trained expert analyzing and interpreting a phylogenic tree. Evolutionary virologists, in their present-day quest to understand how genes "flow" from one host to another and how viruses move through their natural environments, seek not to foretell the future, but to be better prepared in the present. The resultant informational "flow" between labs is thus integral to the scientific pursuit not only of knowledge regarding the origins of circulating and evolving pandemic influenza strains, but also of understanding of their viral natures.

The past is ever present in influenza science. And in more ways than one.

As the "model" virus for the scientific study of disease emergence and evolution (see Morse and Schluederberg 1990 and Webster et al. 1992 for further explication of how influenza came to be paradigmatic for research on other emerging viruses), influenza has been studied for over a century (Webster et al. 1992, 153). In a sense, it is the rich history and long-standing practice of influenza research that connects people, places, and things like viral samples in the present tense; evolutionary virology entails a practice of looking for origins that is only partially captured by the creation and reading of phylogenetic trees. Virus samples are collected; they are shared; they are sequenced collaboratively in a lab;[19] their genetic information is analyzed collaboratively on the web. This material and informational chain intraconnects scientists and interconnects the people, practices, and the objects that they study. This process, in turn, helps to create the expertise that is the driver of the developing superorganism of Global Public Health itself.

Guesstimating the Future

It would be facile to assume that the information generated in the lab about viral RNA is merely a fixation within the epidemiological community. Yet whenever I discussed the matter with epidemiologists or public health officials, it often seemed to me that recent advancements in the quality, speed, and cost of sequencing technology had turned the solution to every problem into a random series of amino acids. As I spent more time with virologists and epidemiologists, however, I began to see that what appeared to be a preoccupation with genetic information and phylogenic trees was not just about our modern fascination with DNA and genetic codes.

If virologists are interested in knowing about the genetic makeup of viruses to better understand viral ecology and evolution, then epidemiologists want to see an analysis of a virus's RNA so that they may make better guesses about the future of a developing pandemic. There is an epistemological rupture between the science in the lab and its application. Virologists and epidemiologists have different interpretations of the same phylogenetic information because they have, in effect, different training and dissimilar goals (though "related" to each other, virology and epidemiology are two very different "families" within global public health). The epidemiologists' "practical" goals of predicting the virus's future actions are more immediate, since they view themselves as front-line fighters in the effort to halt the spread of the virus. They are also under greater political and public pressure to provide answers and issue official recommendations for response.

In the spring of 2009, they sought out those answers, at least partially, by reading articles on the origins of H1N1 comparing the 2009 strain to its deadlier relatives—like the 1918 or 1957 flus. The potential for high transmissibility or severity was, as it were, "all in the family" of H1N1 viruses. One might be able to surmise what the 2009 A(H1N1) virus would be by comparing it to its relatives, or by looking for family resemblances. Biological kinship here holds out a deadly potentiality. Epidemiologists looked to the experts in evolutionary virology to provide them with pertinent clues to deciphering how deadly the 2009 virus *might* be. But, in the end, they had to use their own public health expertise to make sense of the virologists' analyses.

A bevy of scientific articles and analyses of the H1N1 genetic sequences was published during the first few months of the pandemic. In addition to relying upon their own personal experience and other epidemiological and clinical data, the people I worked with had to guess things about the pandemic based upon the phylogenetic tree of H1N1. One clear worry was that the 2009 A(H1N1) virus might be a cousin of the deadlier H5N1—or share some similar avian ancestry. Indeed, all pandemic strains are technically related to "bird flu" (Morens and Taubenberger 2010). The circulating 2009 virus was compared antigenetically to other known strains and determined to be a product of frequent reassortment events (Bhoumik and Hughes 2010). By July 2009, virologists determined that "The likely explanation for the origin of this novel H1N1 influenza virus is that a reassortment event occurred between the North American triple reassortant and the European swine influenza virus" (Brockwell-Staats et al. 2009, 211). What counted for those making decisions concerning pandemic response within epidemiology, however, was that the 2009 virus did not share key characteristics of its deadlier relatives. The phylogenetic tree for the 2009 A (H1N1) virus was shown to have "genetic roots" in the 1918 H1N1 viral strain; the virus that had killed an estimated twenty to forty million people was clearly an "ancestor virus" of the 2009 swine flu (ScienceDaily 2009). What the 2009 virus didn't have, however, were the genetic "markers for virulence that made the 1918 pandemic strain so deadly" (Silberner and Greenfieldboyce 2009). It is this comparison of known markers through time that epidemiologists working "on the ground" during a pandemic are especially eager to lay their hands on in the earliest weeks of a pandemic. For most epidemiologists, then, a virus's past could and would be used to make guesses about the future. More than just a semantic definition of the "future" seems at stake here.

Although virologists like Gavin Smith might warn against using such genetic markers for predictive purposes, most of the public health officials I knew were comfortable basing their own personal predictions on such information, which was consistently viewed as a key part of decision-making during the early days of the outbreak. If the 2009 virus did not show any genetic markers for increased lethality, then less drastic measures could be taken to mitigate the spread of the flu. If, however, the 2009 virus *had* shown marked similarities to its 1918 ancestor, public health authorities would have erred on the side of caution by instituting more drastic containment measures (such as school closures and social distancing) to slow the spread of the pandemic. This "best guesswork" was at the heart of the quiet debates over the uses of phylogenetic trees between evolutionary virologists and their epidemiological counterparts within national and international public health agencies. The virologists were uncomfortable making any sort of predictions based upon the known RNA sequences. As Dr. Ruben Donis, the CDC's chief molecular virologist, stated in an interview for *Science* in May of 2009, the virus might have revealed a part of its complicated evolutionary history, but its RNA alone could not help to answer the question of its specific origins (Cohen 2009b, 701). But the epidemiologists and public health officials, on the other hand, were not so troubled by using such incomplete information to respond to what they saw as a potentially serious threat to public health.

In other words, there was a "natural" limit to what might be conjectured about the virus from information about its gene segments. The virus illuminated the connections between times and places at the same time that it concealed them. One might trace the H1N1 virus's path, but would ultimately be left guessing at its origins. Had a pig farm worker from Canada infected pigs in Mexico with the virus? Had a virus from the United States traveled to Asia through the pig trade? Had birds and pigs come into contact in animal husbandry in Eastern Europe? In a very real sense, such questions regarding the biological origins of an influenza virus remain inherently unanswerable. Yet even if the origins of the 2009 A(H1N1) virus itself remain hazy, what became perfectly clear by "reading" phylogenetic trees was that disparate people, animals, viruses, and locations are all interconnected. The main characteristic of those global connections is, as I will argue further in chapter 6, viral. Expertise and information spread out along the same lines as the routes of virus transmission.

On Origins, Revisited

Phylogeny is crucial to understanding how a novel influenza strain becomes labeled as a pandemic in the first place, as well as vital to unlocking the "origins" of pandemic strains. Sequencing of influenza viruses, and the subsequent construction and analysis of phylogenetic trees, is derivative and productive of viral expertise. The divide between evolutionary virologists and epidemiologists over the interpretation of a virus's phylogeny, as well as the production of meaning about this information, highlights how different groups of scientists enact expertise in real time both during and after a pandemic. The focus on gene flows above mirrors the flows of information between scientists throughout the 2009 H1N1 pandemic.

If biology is one way to begin unpacking the complex origin story of the 2009 H1N1 virus, then geography is another. Historically conceptualized as an epicenter or origin point of infectious diseases, Hong Kong continues to play a significant role in the interpretation and circulation of epidemiological, clinical, and virological information on influenza in the twenty-first century. The following two chapters will explore Hong Kong's role as the "home" of influenza and a global center of scientific research on Influenza A, highlighting how epidemiologists working in the city during 2009 enacted viral expertise through the decision to quarantine.

2

The Invisible Chapter
(Work In the Lab)

The endless cycle of idea and action,
Endless invention, endless experiment,
Brings knowledge of motion, but not of stillness;
Knowledge of speech, but not of silence;
Knowledge of words, and ignorance of the Word.

T. S. Eliot, *The Rock*

Gene Segment PB1. Biological function: *Part of the polymerase complex with PB2 and PA, PB1 aids in transcription. Mutations in this segment can alter a virus's ability to replicate. A variant of this protein, called PB1-F2, is thought to be a determinant of a virus's virulence. Both the H5N1 and 1918 H1N1 strains contained this variant, but the 2009 H1N1 virus lacked it.* Pathographic function: *Part of a "biological narratives complex" with chapter 1, this segment goes inside a laboratory in Hong Kong to examine "routine" scientific work that extracts information about Influenza A viruses from soil and tissue samples. The discovery and genetic sequencing of viruses in a "local" setting is representative of the replication of "universal" or standardized lab protocols. These material practices ground all subsequent knowledge about flu, forming the basis for pandemic response and policy decisions.*

On Material Discourse

Prior to the 2009 H1N1 pandemic, I had no practical experience working in a lab. I hadn't become accustomed to the near-constant whirring of a centrifuge or the patient ticking of an old-fashioned egg timer in an otherwise hushed lab. Hadn't developed any sensory memory of the distinct smell of particular chemicals or the feel of my fingers encased in thin latex gloves. Hadn't ever learned to deftly handle the various instruments or tools: pipettes, Petri dishes, plastic tubes, gel boxes. Hadn't stuffed the large pockets of a white lab coat with various pens and small, bright Post-it notes reminding me to ask follow-up questions about networked fridge monitors or modern methods of virus quantification. In other words, I had little tacit understanding of how the science behind influenza research was actually performed.

My education in all these matters began on a rainy, cold morning in March 2010, when I took a twenty-minute bus ride from my apartment in Central District, Hong Kong, out to the western part of the island. I was on my way to the University of Hong Kong to see Professor Frederick C. Leung, a biologist whose laboratory specializes in the sequencing and scientific analysis of zoonotic viruses. In 2003, Leung had worked on the genetic sequencing of the SARS coronavirus. I knew his name not only from the history of the SARS outbreak, but from his having been a former Ph.D. student at Berkeley. When I first began the hunt for a host institution for fieldwork, Leung had been Berkeley's liaison with HKU. His emails had been warm and enthusiastic and he had offered me assistance not only with my project, but in locating affordable housing (itself a gargantuan task in a city like Hong Kong).

By the time that I took the bus to Fred Leung's lab, the genetic sequencing and analysis of the 2009 A (H1N1) influenza virus had long been completed, but routine surveillance and sequencing of Influenza A subtypes is a perpetual activity. The lab was one of many in the city involved in the ongoing sampling of soil and tissues from live bird markets and surrounding farms in the New Territories and Guangdong Province.

Unlike most of his contemporaries, Leung does not believe that highly pathogenic H5N1 is a pandemic threat to humans, a "heretical" view to which I will return in chapter 7. He believes his vocal support of this view has led him to be ostracized from the rest of the research community in the city. In many ways, then, his lab is both "typical" and "atypical" in regard to the surveillance and study of influenza viruses. Still, as I was repeatedly assured by Leung's diligent postdoctoral fellow, Dr. Raymond Hui, who ran the day-to-day operations of the lab, the techniques I witnessed there would be the same standardized procedures[1] used in the discovery and sequencing of viruses everywhere (including those performed in Robert Webster's lab). The location of individual laboratories and the geographic origin of the virus samples changed, but the scientific practice was always similar. In essence, then, what I would be observing was the discovery and sequencing of the 2009 A (H1N1) influenza virus by proxy.

Raymond was in charge of my time in the lab, and often lamented that most of the things I would have the opportunity to witness were quite dull and repetitive. "But when we find what we expect to find, or what we said we wanted to find," he said, instantly smiling and opening his eyes wider, "that's when this work is really exciting. Then everything we do is worth the effort." But most of the time, Raymond cautioned, we wouldn't find anything all that new or interesting in the samples. On a typical day, it would just be "routine" laboratory activities. The process was "boring" and there was a lot of waiting—for cell cultures to be ready, for DNA replication cycles to complete, for sequencing machines to do their job. I sensed that Raymond was more than a bit perplexed by my strong desire to be in the lab as he silently processed soil samples and sequenced influenza viruses. But it was specifically this routinized, muted, and almost invisible search for influenza viruses and the attendant material practices of the lab that I was interested in observing.

This chapter describes the virological science and the material laboratory practice of looking for and sequencing novel Influenza A viruses. Although the science examined throughout is "universal," this chapter is set in Hong Kong because, and as will be explored in more depth in Chapter 3, laboratories in this particular city are in a uniquely superior position to obtain a steady supply of the necessary samples for influenza surveillance. Turning soil and swab samples into information or knowledge about influenza is a lengthy and hands-on, or embodied, process. In essence, then, this chapter narrates the invisible practices that undergird much of influenza science. Stefan Helmreich suggests in his work on marine biotechnology that laboratory techniques such as the ones I describe below are indistinguishable from "institutional apparatuses" (2009, 106) such as pandemic plans, WHO International Health Regulations, and the CDC's Emergency Operations Center. Even if the specific lab techniques are often unspoken, they form the backbone of everything scientists know—or want to know—about how influenza viruses act in the world outside the laboratory (as we saw in more detail in Chapter 1). Knowing something about the everyday material practices behind the creation of phylogeny trees in evolutionary virology is integral to understanding—more viscerally—how viruses, those who work with or are affected by them, and superorganisms like the emergent global public health network are interrelated.

Following Isabelle Stengers, I examine the scientific paradigm that drives present-day virology as a "way of doing" or "intervening" (2000, 49)—not just as a way of "thinking about" viruses. While observing in Fred Leung's lab I began to think that what virology laboratories were constructing through these material processes was not—reductio ad absurdum—the virus itself, or even simply "knowledge" about a virus, but rather a complex network of scientists, laboratories, farms, public health institutions, and other actors involved in the circulation of influenza samples and genetic information about influenza viruses (a point I explored in Chapter 1 in relationship to phylogenetics). The laboratory, then, might be better conceptualized as constructing a type of relationality between nonliving and living things, between humans and nonhumans, between individuals and social institutions. The standard laboratory techniques that I observed were, in essence, part of the infrastructure of global public health (Lampland and Star 2009). And as scholar Elizabeth Dunn reminds us so poignantly: "Although standards present themselves as *episteme*, as pure idea that exists outside of particular places, standards need an *oikodomi*, a material context in which they are transformed into action and effect" (2009, 120). The material practice of the lab techniques that I examine below transform the influenza virus into an artifact that is "simultaneously *ideal* (conceptual) and material" (Bowker and Star 1999, 289).

Ultimately, the laboratory is the site of a silent orchestral movement with a virus as its invisible conductor. If anthropologist Celia Lowe uses the "cloud" as a metaphor "to indicate the clusters of biosocialities in play and at work with H5N1 in Indonesia" (2010, 627), then I use networks of expertise as a lens for looking at the practices of lab science in Hong Kong. I explore how "touching" the virus, manipulating it, and eventually "reading" it, helps to build social and professional networks. This is perhaps less than surprising, since scholars have already made the claim that standards and infrastructures are really about relationality (Lampland and Star 2009, 17). One must learn these standard lab techniques under the tutelage of other, more experienced, scientists. I was interested too, then, in the lab as a type of relational ecology—an environment that shaped those who worked within it.

What follows is not, however, simply about the construction or representation or symbolic capital of viruses. Akin to Pierre Bourdieu, I push back here against the all too common tendency "to reduce laboratory activity to a semiological activity" or "textism" (2004, 3, 28). The work of the laboratory, in fact, is not entirely about the inscription practices of scientists or their production of scientific articles on viruses. It is about materiality, too, but a material that is "tangible rather than abstract" (Boivin 2010, 25–26). I therefore include all the technological apparatus of the laboratory here as part of the material, or the "scientific things" (Rheinberger 2010, 1) that I want to study as part of the influenza virus and the 2009 H1N1 pandemic itself. Here I re-create the material and technological process of the discovery and sequencing of the lab: its physical techniques, its sense of time, its spaces, its methods, its ennui, and its surprising silences.[2] As the concept of phenomenotechnique suggests, one must understand how knowledge about a scientific object like an influenza virus is produced through the machines and method of their production (Rheinberger 2010, 31).

In other words, it is time to revisit the laboratory without Bruno Latour or Karin Knorr-Cetina or even Harry Collins, but perhaps always already in their significant shadows. Indeed, it is difficult, if not almost impossible, to envision any ethnography of the laboratory without recourse to its social-scientific past. To remedy this, I turn to a poet. Hearkening back to the T. S. Eliot quote that opens this chapter, I am interested in exploring how ideas and actions, inventions and experiments, motion and stillness, and speech and silence interplay within the enclosed and partially "hidden" microbiology laboratory to produce "visible" knowledge about influenza. Ultimately, I hope that understanding how scientists grapple with centrifuges, soil samples, PCR (polymerase chain reaction) machines, and RNA might shed more analytical light on the problematic relationship between theories of material and discourse in social studies of science. This relationship between material and discourse, or *material discourse*, highlights the ways in which the exchange of technology, methods, virus samples—or material—and "discourse" or information about viruses helps to craft and reinforce networks of viral expertise.

A Boring Process Reproduced in Excruciating Detail and Repeated Ad Infinitum

Fred Leung's lab focuses on the study of longitudinal change in the genetic makeup of viruses found in soil samples. The project involves the processing, genetic mapping, and analysis of viruses found in samples collected on a monthly basis from the same livestock farms. It was fortuitous, Leung told me on my first visit with him, that his lab assistants would return from one of the farms the weekend before I was scheduled to observe inside the lab. I would have the chance to observe the entire process from start to finish—from soil sample to RNA to data on a computer.

The particular samples I would be helping to process had been collected with sterile cotton swabs from soil surrounding a central pond and in randomly selected locations throughout a farm located in Guangdong Province. After collection, the samples were deposited in clear plastic test tubes with a transport material; the tubes were then packed in ice and sealed inside a white Styrofoam cooler in order to preserve any biological organisms. The practice of collecting and transporting viral samples, I quickly realized, was the first instantiation of how material or biological objects could connect disparate people and locations into a common network. The free collection of samples required a delicate balance between researcher and farmer. These personal relationships, developed over time and built on trust between particular farmers and particular researchers, had bled into the routine collection of samples. The practice had—over time—crafted a relationship or bond between farmers and scientists. Fred Leung, in particular, felt a strong allegiance to the farmers; he had promised to never divulge their identity or location to the authorities, despite the fact that he was often pressed to do so.

But soil samples do not just help to craft relationships between scientists and farmers. Samples are also the raw material that must be turned into knowledge. Feces and dirt are the stuff of science. They are the first instantiation of the material objects with which the scientist must come into relationship. As science studies scholar Karen Knorr-Cetina has noted, laboratories "install reconfigured scientists who become workable (feasible) in relation to these objects." The lab is thus a "workshop and a nursery" for nurturing and intervening; biological objects in the lab are "processing materials." Laboratories like Leung's are spaces that reconfigure the relationships between "self-other-things." (Knorr-Cetina 1999, 29, 37.)

It is the "boring" process of turning soil samples into information about influenza viruses that reconfigures the relationship of the scientists to their object of study. Bringing the soil samples into the lab is, in essence, similar to what Callon, Lascoumes, and Barthes label "Translation 1." The world—or the macrocosm—is "transported" into the laboratory so that it may be dealt with as part of a microcosm. But as Callon et al. point out, "what is in the laboratory is at once different and similar" (2009, 50) to what is found in the so-called real world. The materiality of the soil must be transformed in some way in order for scientists to work with it. It is this process of transformation that I detail immediately below.

Part One—Discovery

The first step in the process assumes as its foundational premise that each soil sample is "positive" for virus: all samples are initially presumed to contain live viruses of some indeterminate nature. That means, in essence, that all samples will be tested for confirmation of the presence of viruses. Should a sample then be confirmed as positive for the presence of influenza through the PCR process, that virus will be replicated in cultured cells and its RNA genetically sequenced and compared to those of other known viruses.

Building on the work of philosopher John Searle, it becomes crucial to point out here that the viruses in the soil samples are both institutional and brute facts at this stage. Even if the virus as a fact is "observer-relative" or "ontologically subjective" throughout the testing and sequencing process, that does not mean that the virus cannot also be viewed as a "natural" physical or material object that exists outside of virus-human interaction. There is a difference, as Searle suggests, between *constructing* objects to serve a human purpose and *assigning a function* to naturally occurring objects. Therefore, I assume throughout this narrative retelling of scientific practice, that viruses are constitutive of both "agentive functions"—or intentional uses given to objects by humans—and "nonagentive functions"—or functions that remain independent of the "practical intentions and activities of human agents." (Searle 1995, 10, 14, 20.) It is vital to view viruses in relationship to this interstitial position in order to effectively analyze what agentive functions or "work" they do as the foundation of a multibillion-dollar global research paradigm. Pushing the idea of "agency" of objects like the influenza virus further, anthropologist Jane Bennett creates a theoretical space to talk about a "vital materiality" or "vital materialism" of things. By "vitality," Bennett simply means the "capacity of things . . . not only to impede or block the will and designs of humans but also to act as quasi agents or forces with trajectories, propensities, or tendencies of their own." She relies upon Spinoza's concept of "conatus," or the active "tendency to persist" that is a property of every body—human and nonhuman alike—to make a case that material things are "associative" in that they are always affecting and being affected by each other. (Bennett 2010, viii, 2, 21.) In this case, the scientists, the soil samples, and the viruses are all affecting and being affected by each other. In some ways, this is a co-constitutive process, as Knorr-Cetina hints when she suggests that scientists themselves are "methods of inquiry; they are part of a field's research strategy and a technical device in the production of knowledge" (1999, 29).

Once I don a borrowed white lab coat and store my things under one of the work benches in the main lab, Raymond guides me toward Leung's Biosafety Level 2 (BSL-2) laboratory. We pass through a series of two heavy doors, separated by a short hallway cluttered with metal storage cabinets, and into an average-sized room. The room itself is painted white and packed with equipment: refrigerators; large, standing tanks that I presume contain some kind of gas; a few black swivel chairs scattered at the workbenches; rows of boxes that contain tubes, pipette covers, rubber gloves; a set of stainless-steel sinks; and, the most important piece of equipment in the room, a hooded (or ventilated) workbench.

Almost instantly, I realize that I am in a room *that contains viruses*. I feel nervous for a moment before my anxiety dissipates into intense excitement. I have read about and studied potentially deadly viruses for years, but I have never *seen* any of them. It is almost like preparing to meet a favorite celebrity; I experience a fan's sense of nervous anticipation and delight.

Raymond opens the door of a midsized cabinet to take out a small, clear plastic tray of cell cultures. Viruses need to replicate within host cells; scientists essentially use cancerous cells (which are themselves known for their ability to replicate) to propagate and study viral samples. All cell cultures are kept in an incubator stationed inside the BSL-2 area of the lab at exactly 35.2°C and 5% CO_2, Raymond explains, because this temperature and CO_2 percentage are the optimum levels for preserving and culturing viruses. The tray in Raymond's outstretched hand looks similar to an ice tray or a watercolor tray—with tiny wells in rows. Raymond points to the configuration of cells, eight down by ten across, and explains that each column contains the same dilution of virus, with each row containing a different dilution. Eight samples, then, are at exactly the same dilution of virus (the purpose of repetition being to provide a control for the statistical variability inherent in a biological process like viral replication). Different dilutions, Raymond explains, are used to calculate the $TCID_{50}$ for virus titer (or the concentration level of the virus that will lead to infection in 50 percent of inoculated cells). As he is explicating terms for me, Raymond carefully tapes the cell culture tray with a thin plastic film so that we will be able to transport the tray outside the BSL-2 area of the lab. The tape will trap any viruses inside the tray, preventing contamination outside of the BSL-2 area.

"I prepared this earlier for you, so you could see a good result. I already knew that there was virus in the sample I used to culture these," Raymond says as he leads me back out to the main lab, threading his way to a set of microscopes at a workstation. He tell me he wants me to see for myself what an infected cell looks like. As he places the tray under the microscope, I am almost giddy. It is the closest I will get, without benefit of an electron microscope, to seeing a virus. I can't actually see the virus, but what I can observe are the direct cellular effects that indicate its existence.

I take off my glasses and peer through the lens at the cell inside the tray well. As I do so, Raymond interprets what I am viewing. First, he has me look at a negative sample—one without any evidence of virus. The uninfected cell resembles a series of light, banded lines in a trapezoidal shape. Then Raymond repositions the tray and instructs me to look again, this time at a positive sample—at a cell showing evidence of virus. Even as a novice, I note the difference. Whereas an uninfected cell is visualized as straight lines, an infected cell has a more rounded appearance. Raymond calls this a "display of detachment" (or evidence of cell degeneration). Evidence of detachment is the cytopathic effect (CPE) used to calculate the $TCID_{50}$.

It is important to fully admit that I had never heard the terms $TCID_{50}$ or CPE before Raymond first uttered them in the lab. Presuming I had at least a basic knowledge of virology, Raymond used specific scientific terminology as a matter of course. I had to stop him in midsentence several times, at least initially, so that I might be able to grasp everything he said. I scribbled words and acronyms down in my notebook as fast as possible while still trying to listen intently. Apprentice where Raymond was expert, I rued not having taken any introductory microbiology classes. Everything was new and exciting for me; for Raymond, however, these procedures were already rote. He was clearly operating on an embodied "lab autopilot," and I noticed him straining to slow down, to move more deliberately and consciously through all the routine steps involved in "finding" a virus in a soil sample, to carefully explain the minutiae of the material processes to me. After I—finally—began to understand some of the terms myself, I felt elated. It was incredible to see an influenza virus, or rather, to see the effects of the virus on a cell. It occurred to me that I was a witness in the scientific process of detecting a virus, isolating it, seeing its visible effects, and then sequencing it—all in a collective effort to make its origins "readable." The laboratory, à la Latour and Woolgar (1979) or Shapin and Schaffer (1985), really did make the invisible visible.

But it did something else, too. In Callon's terms, such "inscription" is indicative of the "research collective at work" in what he terms Translation 2. Callon argues that "The inscription is infralinguistic. It is an inducement to talk." Here, "traces" of viruses in soil samples become interwoven with statements about them; the lab itself is conceived as an enormous inscription device. Scientific knowledge is embodied here. Raymond had difficulty explaining things to me as he was doing them because of the tacit knowledge required to practice science. He slowed his movements so that I could capture what he was doing. I was not so much learning as absorbing information through a pas de deux between talk and doing, between discourse and material. Callon argues that "The most theoretical science always sinks its roots in the material and bodily practices that informed it and without which it could not be put to work and enriched." More importantly, this type of practice and knowledge is "10 percent explicit and codified and 90 percent tacit and embodied—embodied in instruments (Bachelard: 'Instruments are only materialized theories. They produce phenomena that bear the stamp of theory on every side'), in disciplined bodies, in purified substances, in reagents, in laboratory animals (like Drosophilia, or a transgenic mouse), or even in reference materials." (Callon et al. 2009, 51, 54, 55.)

The entire scientific process for manipulating viral material in soil samples is both painstaking and precise. It requires skill and practice in order to carry it out effectively, to produce "good" results or "good" theory. In essence, the steps that I observed in Fred Leung's lab produced the virus as a concrete or material object that could subsequently be examined, studied, and further manipulated. The material process for extracting viral RNA from samples and then "amplifying" them so that they could be genetically sequenced was even more lengthy, and took repeat visits to the lab to observe from beginning to end. In what follows, I re-create the repetitive nature and ennui of the process through an exacting description of the physical steps necessary to produce enough viral material for sequencing. My point is to mimic these material processes in the present tense for the reader, so that he or she may visualize and virtually—and viscerally—experience the lab.

Part Two—Discovery (*continued*)

Step one is to add a chemical reagent called TRIzol to soil samples in the test tubes. At this stage, we are only processing a small part of a sample, and can come back to the remainder if the results are positive. Reagents are substances added to chemical reactions or systems to produce, detect, or to measure other substances. In this case, TRIzol is a popular reagent used to isolate genetic material from tissue or cell samples. After adding TRIzol, the samples can be safely transported out of the BSL-2 lab, as the reagent completely breaks down any viruses in the soil without damaging the genetic material. Handheld pipettes, the size of a very large marker, are used to transfer small amounts of liquid between tiny vessels. Plastic barrier pipette tips are used to prevent contamination during the process. I watch as Raymond uses a new tip for each separate sample, adding to the length of time he has to spend working under the ventilation hood. His almost mechanical actions have the additional effect of making the BSL-2 area seem eerily reminiscent of a factory production line.

TRIzol, Raymond explains as he works, can extract both RNA (typically from a virus though bacteria also have RNA) and DNA (usually indicative of bacteria, but some viruses also have DNA instead of RNA) from the sample, making it an excellent reagent for use in detecting unknown microorganisms. Once the reagent has been added, Raymond packs each tube in ice. Because RNA is easily degraded, he clarifies, it is "best practice" to keep the samples cool at all times.

Back in the main area of the lab, Raymond adds chloroform to the reagent mixture. Each tube is then vortexed for exactly ten seconds. When a tube is pressed against a vortex machine, it vibrates at a high speed, reminiscent of the way a sonic toothbrush operates. Effectively, vortexing is a method of mixing viscous liquid materials in a "wet lab."[3] Vortexing produces a different quality of "mixture" than does merely "shaking" the tube. When vortexed, the mixture inside the tube transforms from a clear pink to an opaque pink in color and is then incubated for exactly three minutes.

Raymond sets a kitchen timer and we chat about life in the lab, about how interesting he finds his work, about how Hong Kong is the best place to do research on viruses (see chapter 3). After three minutes, we walk the tubes over to a centrifuge, and run the machine at 12,000 × g for ten minutes. Our chatting continues. I notice that it is difficult for Raymond to both talk to me and work with the materials. Talking distracts him and he often pauses in order to think about his explanations of what is, for him, routine work. For Bourdieu, such embodied practice is evidence of a "scientific habitus" as "realized, embodied theory" (2004, 40). Raymond's inability to articulate the reasons behind his actions is proof of the limits of discourse about material processes in the lab. Nothing is being inscribed in the procedures; Raymond is not even keeping detailed notes of what he is doing at this stage of the process. Because nothing, as it were, is remarkable or notable to him.[4] As Bourdieu suggests: "When they [scientists] try to express their sense of correct procedure, they have little to call on beyond their past experience, which remains implicit and quasi-corporeal, and when they talk informally about their research, they describe it as a practice requiring experience, intuition, skill, flair, a 'knack,' all things difficult to set down on paper, which can only really be understood and acquired by example and through personal contact with competent persons" (2004, 39). What I was witnessing in Fred Leung's lab was nothing more and nothing less than the result of years of past experience, corporealized.[5] Raymond was providing me with material examples so that I might enter further into the discourse about viruses. His competence would, hopefully, rub off on me. To use a term from Collins and Evans (2009), I was gaining a type of "interactional expertise" during my time with Raymond. Interactional expertise is "the bridge between full-scale physical immersion in a form of life (which gives rise to contributory expertise) and non-expert acquaintanceship with the idea of [skill] and the discourse pertaining to it" (59). If I was not "of" the lab, then I could become acquainted intimately enough with it to become "quasi-expert" myself.

Post-centrifuge, the mixture in each test tube visibly separates out into three distinct layers. I note how each step in the material processing of samples produces clear visual changes inside the tube. The pink bottom layer, Raymond says as he points out the thick-looking substance gathered at the bottom of the tube, holds any DNA that viruses or bacteria in the sample may have contained. A thin white film on top of the DNA layer is the protein layer. Raymond explains that the protein layer might be much thicker, depending on the type of transport medium used and the amount of organisms in the sample (transport medium is a substance used to preserve a biological sample until it reaches the lab). At the very top of the tube is a clear, watery layer, or "aqueous phase," that contains what we are looking for—RNA. The RNA separates from the rest of the mixture due to differences in solubility (the ability of a substance to be dissolved in a solvent).

At this stage, Raymond begins the process of collecting the upper aqueous phase into a clean test tube. While he is doing this, I take pictures over his shoulder. Raymond stresses that the pipette should not touch the other material layers inside the tube; if it does, it will contaminate—and ruin—the experiment. I watch as Raymond collects all the aqueous phase that is possible without touching the pipette tip to the protein layer. In different experiments, the process might be much more difficult, Raymond explains. If he is looking for mRNA (or messenger RNA), then the aqueous phase is even thinner

Midway through, Raymond suddenly offers to let me try pipetting out the aqueous phase. He holds the pipette out to me and I quickly demur. Then we both laugh.

"It takes practice," he says. "Most students have no pipetting skill at first. We try to collect as much as possible because we don't know the virus titer [the concentration of virus]—if it's low, then we'll need as much as possible."

Part Three—Amplification

Raymond then adds isopropanol to each tube and explained that this step is for the "precipitation of the RNA particles"—a process that concentrates the viral RNA even when few viruses are present. (Precipitation in chemistry refers to the formation of a substance from a solution, or of a solid from a liquid.) After the samples are incubated for ten minutes,

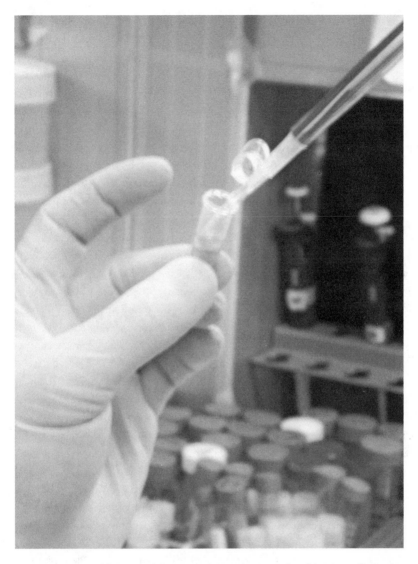

Figure 4. A display of dexterity. After ten years of experience in a virology lab, Raymond's pipetting skill was almost flawless. Daily practice is part of a series of techniques required for success in the lab, forming part of a "habitus" of laboratory work.

they are placed back in the centrifuge for another ten-minute spin. The "supernatant"—or the liquid that remains "floating" above a substance after precipitation and/or centrifugation—is then simply poured out of each tube into a collection tub at the work station for waste disposal.

Remaining at the bottom of the tube is a white RNA pellet. Raymond explains that the samples we are processing have produced a particularly big RNA pellet, and that sometimes the pellet from other samples is so small that it will not be visible to the naked eye. "But even if it isn't visible," Raymond explains, "we assume the RNA pellet is there." A solution (EtOH— or alcohol) is then added to the pellet to remove any salt. The tube is given another "short spin," and the additional supernatant is aspirated (all the liquid is removed). After this, once again only the RNA pellet remains at the bottom of the tube. Finally, water is added to the tube to "resuspend" the RNA pellet. Each tube is then individually vortexed to dissolve the pellet. This is where viral RNA extraction ends, and where the process of complementary DNA (cDNA) synthesis begins.

I want to pause our narrative here to briefly discuss the concept of synthesis. At this stage of the material processing of viral samples, more genetic material must be produced—or the viral genome must be amplified— before the virus can be genetically sequenced. This is the physical beginning of what will eventually become information about a virus's genetic makeup and its genetic phylogeny. From the perspective of actor-network theory, developed by Latour, Callon, and others, the virus here is an "actant" (itself a term used, in part, to move away from the divide between subjects and objects, humans and nonhumans). What is important in the theory is the *interaction* between humans and nonhumans and the networks that develop as a result of this human/nonhuman interface. This requires, Latour argues, that we "rethink anew the role of objects in the construction of collectives" (1993, 55). Here I also want to insert Searle's suggestion that biology and culture are not oppositional, but fused, and that "culture is the form that biology takes" (1995, 227). What Latour and Searle are both arguing, albeit from different standpoints, is that there is a continuum between the ontology of biology and the ontology of cultural or institutional forms.

I argued in chapter 1 that the network of virologists, epidemiologists, public health officials, and various other "actants" is born out of, as it were, the biology of the influenza virus. As such, the network mirrors the characteristics and functions of the virus. Philosopher Karen Barad's concept of "agential realism" suggests that it is the "intra-action" of object and human that produces the scientific object—in this case, viral RNA. Her use of the term intra-action is an avowed attempt to move beyond the dichotomy of subject and object, suggesting instead that the object and the subject's "observation" of it are indissoluble (Barad 1999, 5). In other words, the virus being synthesized and genetically sequenced is *indistinguishable* from the scientist's grasp of it. The RNA pellet, then, is a type of "vital materialism" (Bennett 2010) or "reified theorem" (Bachelard, quoted in Rheinberger 2011). The technology that is used to produce RNA is inseparable from the scientist who processes the samples. Everything becomes "amplified" through the material processing of the laboratory.

Part Four—How to Culture a Virus

Back in the BSL-2 area of the lab, Raymond switches gears to show me what happens if samples are positive for virus. First, saline is added to the sample and it is filtered in order to "sterilize" it. This step is referred to as such, Raymond explains, even though the RNA virus itself is kept intact or "viable." The samples must be sterilized before the virus mixture can be added to the cell culture. To do this, the virus mixture is filtered with what looks like a small, blue kitchen sieve with a 0.2 micrometer filter (small enough that most bacteria cannot pass through).

After filtering, the mixture is added to Madin-Darby Canine Kidney epithelial cells for culturing. MDCK cells are regularly used in the amplification of Influenza A viruses due to their permissivity to influenza virus replication. Because of this, they are also being used by some vaccine manufacturers to produce influenza vaccines. To amplify the virus, and before it can be sequenced, a culture medium is added to the MDCK cells mixed with the virus samples to, as Raymond explains, "maintain the pH condition [the acidity or alkaline level of a solution] and to provide nutrients to the cell The culture medium is bright pink, and I find myself briefly pondering why the color pink seems so pervasive in the these experiments.

Raymond dumps the medium out into a collection jar and taps the Petri dish onto a paper towel on his right, performing all of these manipulations under the ventilation hood. He rinses the Petri dish with a saline solution to get rid of any metabolic waste from the cells that might inhibit virus proliferation. After blotting, he adds the virus to the dish. To the untrained eye, the Petri dish looks empty—or perfectly clear. I have to simply trust that the cells are there, clinging to the bottom of the Petri dish, since

I cannot not see them with the naked eye. Wittgenstein's postulation that all certainty is subjective (1969, 33e) flashes through my mind.

Raymond explains that a large volume of virus is never added to the Petri dish because this would reduce an individual virus's chance of infecting a cell. Therefore, only a small amount of virus is added to the dish. The Petri dish is then placed into an incubator for up to two hours. After incubation, another 10 ml of fresh culture medium is added to foster virus growth in the cells. Finally, the culture is placed back into the incubator for five days. Four to five days is enough time, Raymond explains, for the virus to grow and for the cells to show cytopathic effect.

Time seems to flow unevenly within the lab. There are moments when things speed up and long hours or days when all one is doing is waiting. It is the waiting that seems to be the source of the ennui that Raymond (and indeed almost everyone I've ever known who has toiled in a wet lab) warned me about and with which he has found methods to cope. He takes the time that viruses are "culturing" to read articles, go through his notes on the series of experiments, have meetings with Leung and the graduate students under his care. He works on his computer, answering emails or reading the news. He passes time while the viruses replicate inside cells. The viruses are, in this moment, in charge of the tempo of things. They assert their agency over time; they cannot be rushed nor slowed down. Patience is a prerequisite for this type of work. Turning material into information takes time.

Part Five—Ascertaining the $TCID_{50}$

After the virus has been cultured, the next step is to dilute the viral samples in order to ascertain at what dilution 50 percent of the cells exhibit CPE. This information is then used to calculate the $TCID_{50}$ for the virus. The tray itself is rinsed with saline to reduce cell waste (with each well having initially contained MDCK cells and medium), and the virus is applied to cell surfaces with 20 ml of virus solution added to each well. Wells in the control row contain pure medium (without virus). Each dilution of the same sample is carefully labeled by Raymond with –1 through –10. Minus 1 stands for a concentration of 10 × dilution, or 270 ml of saline. The next column is labeled –2, pipetted from the original sample into another well with 270 ml for a 100 × dilution, and so forth.

Diluting the virus, Raymond works back from the lowest to the highest concentration because he wants to utilize the same pipette tip. Doing this in reverse would ruin the dilution and "screw up" the $TCID_{50}$ results. As I watch over his shoulder, he makes at least two errors—or near-errors— when adding the solution to the wells. It is nearly impossible for either one of us to keep track or to tell if a mistake has really been made; the already filled wells show only a light pink color from the medium and are almost indiscernible from the clear, empty wells.

After he is done, Raymond places the tray in the incubator for another two hours. Then, using a vacuum that funnels off residual material through a bleach solution to kill any leftover virus, Raymond suctions off the medium from each well in the tray. The tray is then rinsed with saline to get rid of any unassociated virus particles (or viruses that have not attached themselves to the surface of the cells), which might throw off the results. At this point, most of the viruses have merely attached to the cell surface, but have not yet penetrated the cell wall. The tray needs to be incubated for only two hours because Raymond does not want the

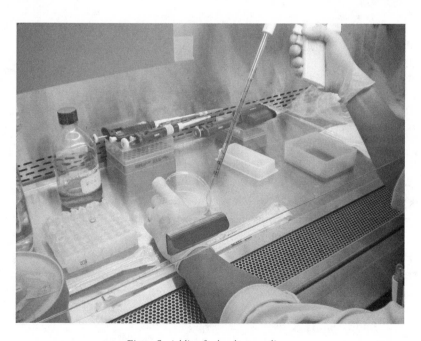

Figure 5. Adding fresh culture medium.

cells to become infected at this stage, as that might negatively affect the attachment rate for other viruses. Raymond explains that once a virus has penetrated a cell, the virus alters the cell's makeup to make it more difficult for other viruses to attach to or penetrate the cell. In essence, Raymond is describing viral competition for available resources.

After the two hours, the wells are suctioned once more after being rinsed with saline. Raymond then adds more culture medium and places the tray back into the incubator for another four or five days. During this time he is waiting for the cells to become infected by a virus, as that will produce the cytopathic effect he is hoping to observe in order to calculate the $TCID_{50}$.

The end result of this procedure is a cell tray with rows and columns of wells similar to the one that I originally looked at under the microscope on my first day observing in the lab. I have, as it were, come full circle in my observational cycle. I am back at the point where I started, and I begin to experience a bit of the monotony inherent to all routine laboratory work. Once the trays are incubated, each well is checked and the results are depicted on a chart.

Part Six—Reverse Transcription

In order to do anything further with the RNA viruses, they have to be turned into DNA through a process of reverse transcription. This process takes place in a PCR machine, interchangeably referred to as a thermocycler.[6] A special reagent mixture (a composite of two DNA primers) is added to the viral RNA (or the end product of the process of RNA extraction above), using the DNA primers as a template for the PCR machine. Two different primers are used during this RT-PCR reaction to reduce any chance of false negatives. Sometimes even when using two primers, Raymond explains, he will still get a negative result. If there is no "PCR hit," there may still be an influenza virus present in the sample, but it will be something unknown or very rare. Using two primers, however, usually insures that he gets a "hit."

During the time I observe him, Raymond processes eight different samples, plus a positive and a negative control sample. The positive control is a "known entity" that produces a specific band of DNA. The negative control is a reagent mixed with water. This is an important step because the positive and negative controls confirm if the reaction has worked (i.e. when there are no positives from samples, but the positive control still shows a positive result), or if there was a possible contamination (i.e. when everything shows a positive result and the negative sample also shows a

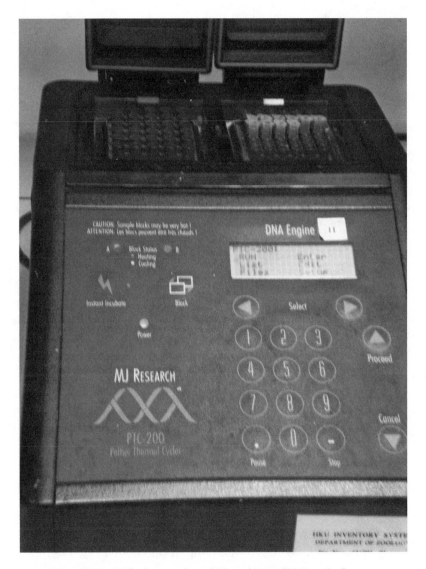

Figure 6. The thermocycler, or PCR machine, or "DNA engine."

positive result). After adding reagent to each sample, Raymond adds a single drop of mineral oil to each tube to protect against evaporation during the temperature fluctuation in the PCR machine. Raymond then explains that thermocyclers usually have a preheat function to help prevent evaporation, but that Fred Leung has found that oil is more effective in preventing evaporation.

After preparation, the samples are placed back in the incubator at 42°C for fifty minutes. The final tubes with samples and reagent mixture are then placed into the thermocycler.

Raymond explains that there are different phases to each "run" in the thermocycler. In phase one, the tubes are heated to 94°C for two minutes to activate the enzymes in the reagent. In phase two, the tubes are kept at 94° for ten seconds to allow the primers to bond with the corresponding sequences in the sample (if the desired DNA is present in the sample). In phase three, the temperature is lowered to 55° for ten seconds to attach the primer to the DNA template. In phase four, the temperature is raised back up to 72° for ten seconds to "turn on" the enzyme that synthesizes a new stretch of DNA. Steps two through five are then repeated for a total of thirty-five complete cycles. In the very last cycle, the samples are kept at 72° for ten minutes to allow the enzyme to fill in any gaps in the newly synthesized DNA strands. After this step, the thermocycler holds the samples at 4°C until the operator removes the samples for further testing. The length of time it takes to complete an entire run depends on the length of the DNA product. The particular runs I observed took approximately one and a half hours to complete. The thermocycler is fully automated; once a run is started it can proceed without any intervention from the operator.

It was at this point in my lab edification that I began to think seriously about Bourdieu's argument, expressing an idea akin to Bachelard's, that "it is the instrument that leads" (2004, 40). So much of the processing of soil samples into information about viruses was about the scientists' understanding of and relationship with the various instruments and machines. Laboratory equipment and humans merged into a working whole. At times, when the machines were whirring or humming it sounded like the low murmur of hushed voices. The quiet in the laboratory, when Raymond and the other lab workers were silently moving about the varied apparatuses, was like the end of all talking and the beginning of all embodied making. The relationships between the soil samples and the viruses, the viruses and the instruments, the instruments and the scientists, and finally, the viruses and the scientists were all intimately bound up in each other. Watching Raymond work, it was clear that "A scientist [really] is a scientific field made flesh" (Bourdieu 2004, 41). The scientist, like the virus, exists materially and ideologically in the laboratory. It is amidst the machines that viruses and scientists are united together to produce the field of virology. The silent, hidden, routine practices are at the heart of everything that we know about influenza. Once established, these routine laboratory methods are usually not discussed further; however, understanding these methods is a key prerequisite to participating in the scientific dialogue. These processes undergird all shared scientific knowledge about influenza. These embodied, rote practices are at the core of the larger networks of viral expertise.

Part Seven—Gel Electrophoresis

After the PCR reactions are completed, a tiny portion of each sample is run through an agarose gel with an electrical current to visualize the results of the reactions. Green dye is added to the samples. Raymond carefully pipettes a few microliters from each tube collected from the PCR machine, making sure to go through the oil layer to the DNA layer beneath, and mixes each sample with green dye in order to "visualize" the PCR product in the gel. The positive and negative controls are also run alongside the samples. For reference, Raymond places a molecular marker in between the sample and control wells, which contains a number of DNA strands of defined lengths.

Each sample is carefully added to a well in the gel itself. I snap a few photos of the wells, but I cannot capture accurately just how tiny they are. A steady hand and excellent pipetting skills are a must at this stage, otherwise, the gel electrophoresis results will be compromised. I am nervous just watching Raymond pipette the samples into the gel.

An electrical current is run through the gel for forty-five minutes, time enough to allow the DNA molecules (which themselves carry a positive charge) to "migrate" through the gel. After electrophoresis, the gel is then stained with ethidium bromide—a highly carcinogenic chemical—that binds onto the DNA molecules. Raymond then places the gel, using a common kitchen spatula, into a "gel dock," and exposes the stained DNA

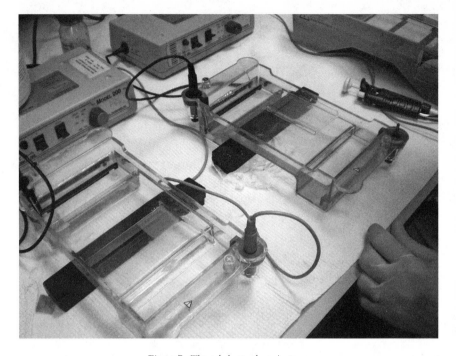

Figure 7. The gel electrophoresis stage.

to ultraviolet light, which can then be visualized and captured via scanner. Raymond reminisces that when he first began to work in a microbiology lab, they still used Polaroid pictures in this step. He is happy that everything has since been digitized. In examining the gel, the samples are compared to the molecular marker, and one turns out to be positive. All positive viral samples in Leung's lab are then sent for DNA sequencing.

Part Eight—DNA Sequencing

The DNA sequencer is located one flight down from Fred Leung's lab in the same university building, housed in a secure, coded-entry room. Raymond tells me that it usually takes about one and a half hours to sequence eight hundred base pairs, but that sixteen separate samples can be run concurrently to save time. Raymond also explains that Professor Leung likes to sequence the full genome of most positive samples, because he believes that a better understanding of viruses can be had by doing so, rather than by just sequencing certain genes or gene segments of a virus—which was still standard practice at the time in most other labs.

When I ask Raymond what his favorite part of the entire process is, he replies: "Getting results that fit your hypothesis is the most satisfying, but

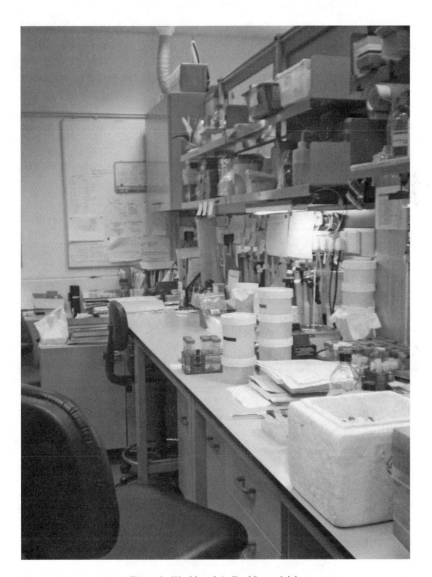

Figure 8. Workbench in Fred Leung's lab.

it only happens in about 20 to 30 percent of the experiments. The rest—the failures, so to speak—are used to restructure our hypothesis. But it is nice when you see what you expect to see."

When I asked Raymond whether or not it is difficult to get farmers to understand the lab's work and to collaborate in the collection of various types of virus samples, he nods. It had been difficult to convince farmers in the New Territories to allow regular sampling, but after the outbreaks of SARS and H5N1 avian influenza, the surveillance has become enforced as a legal mandate. It is far more difficult, Raymond explains, to collect samples from farms on the mainland.

Fred Leung described the situation to me during one of our conversations; the only reason farmers allowed him to regularly collect samples is that the exact location of the farms is concealed. "They trust us," he said. "We understand that they don't want their livestock to be slaughtered. Over the years, we have developed this good relationship with the farmers, so they let us collect our samples."

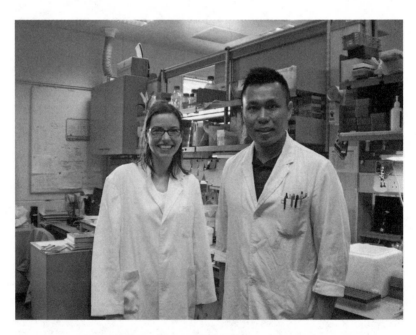

Figure 9. Doctor Raymond Hui and his mostly inept trainee.

The virus samples connect otherwise disconnected individuals and locations. The relationship between the farmers and the scientists in Hong Kong was frequently described to me as "close" and as necessarily "familiar." The exchange of material and useful information prompted a feeling of trust to develop. Particular farms were seen as working with particular labs in a type of trust-based relationship. The materiality of the virus samples was being transformed into a type of relationality built upon the virus itself. The end product of a laboratory in Hong Kong—genetic information on influenza viruses—was only the starting material for the global public health network, where sequences circulated widely and expanded the concept of kinship to include other labs, other farms, other institutions, and other countries.

From the Universal to the Local

Everything we know about flu starts in a lab. The scientific processes explored here form the basis for our larger epidemiological understanding about influenza pandemics and the effectiveness of global public health response actions. In fact, we practice influenza science not just to know, but to affect change in the world. The laboratory is a site where ideas are action, where interventions in the material world take the form of experiments, where motion and stillness intertwine in the habitus of routine lab work, where "textism" comes up against the hard obstacle of stubborn materiality and the "thingness" of viruses. It is a transformative place, which is why so many reams of paper have been spent trying to get at the core of what happens there. Laboratories matter (pun intended), even when they remain silent or invisible to the public eye. Indeed, they are foundational to the larger narratives surrounding influenza.

Historian Roger Hart (1999) has argued that as scholars we must begin to seriously analyze the ways in which certain scientific artifacts—such as the flu virus or techniques of influenza research, surveillance, and control—have become the province of certain cultures, and examine what role such claims may play in the development and creation of those same cultures. This chapter has been an exploration of the universal practice of science in a specific locality—Hong Kong. In the next chapter, I pay attention to the ways in which debates about the local meaning or interpretation of influenza science, especially in relationship to the effectiveness of quarantine, help to recraft much older national and cultural boundaries, despite the increasing effects of globalization and the WHO's attendant attempts to universalize epidemiological response. Nations do not necessarily recede in the face of globalization; rather, governmental and local institutions simply retrench and reconfigure what it means to be "Chinese" or "Hong Kongers" during an influenza pandemic.

3

QUARANTINE, EPIDEMIOLOGICAL KNOWLEDGE, AND INFECTIOUS DISEASE RESEARCH IN HONG KONG

History that repeats itself turns to farce. But a farce that repeats itself ends up making a history.

JEAN BAUDRILLARD, *The Agony of Power*

Gene Segment PA. Biological function: *The polymerase acidic (PA) protein gene is thought to play a key role in the overall virulence of every strain of influenza virus. The segment also plays a pivotal role in the "genome packaging" process, ensuring that each copy of a virus contains a complete copy of all eight gene segments.* Pathographic function: *This segment of the pathography moves us from the realm of virology into that of epidemiology and highlights how local history and geography matter to the enactment of viral expertise. Historical, social, and cultural narratives about Hong Kong as a site for disease outbreaks and research will show us how time and place matter in the construction of knowledge and the evaluation of universal best practices for global pandemic response. In other words, we will see how virological science gets "packaged" and interpreted in relationship to Hong Kong's unique historical, political, and cultural context.*

The Home of Influenza and Expertise

In March 2013, reports of a novel and deadly "bird flu" outbreak in China went viral. The Influenza A subtype at the center of the mounting media attention, H7N9, had never been known to infect humans. Typically, strains of H7N9 are found only in birds. Experts heretofore had remained uncertain about whether or not circulating avian influenzas, such as H7N9 or H9N2, would develop the capacity to regularly infect humans, or, cross-over into a new host. But then the virus effectively jumped the species divide, infecting 132 people[1] and killing 37 (new lab-confirmed cases were still being sporadically reported to the WHO as of this writing). After the outbreak was detected, Chinese authorities randomly tested domestic birds and culled thousands of chickens, ducks, geese, and pigeons in live markets across the country in a concerted effort not only to locate the virus's origin, but to contain the growing outbreak. As epidemiological and clinical details emerged, virologists in China quickly sequenced H7N9. Experts everywhere then began the painstaking process of analyzing the virus's genetic makeup in order to unravel the dual mysteries of where H7N9 had come from and how such a low-path virus (one that barely sickens the birds it infects) had evolved into a strain capable of infecting and killing humans. Just as with H1N1 in 2009 (see chapter 1), genetic information about H7N9 in 2013 was deemed crucial both to predicting what the virus might do and for taking adequate public health measures to halt its spread.

During the initial outbreak, as I exchanged text messages and emails with scientist friends and pored over the information on H7N9 being circulated through Pro-MED (a popular and free internet-based infectious disease reporting service), I experienced a sensation of déjà vu. The 2013 H7N9 outbreak seemed eerily reminiscent of the infamous 1997 outbreak of H5N1 in Hong Kong—an outbreak with which everyone who studies influenza is already very familiar. And unlike in 2009, when H1N1 emerged in Mexico, no one was particularly surprised when a deadlier, if less transmissible, novel strain appeared in China.

China has long been conceptualized as the natural home of influenza. Until 2009, pandemics were, generally speaking, thought to originate in Southeast Asia generally or in China specifically—particularly in subtropical regions such as Guangdong Province. While there is evidence for this,[2] casting China as a primary origin point for most, if not all, novel influenza strains is problematic.[3] For one, influenza viruses circulate in wild birds, which migrate globally. The ability of Influenza A subtypes to mutate inside their avian hosts is not, then, confined to one geographic location. The somewhat popular viewpoint that the animal husbandry practices of Chinese farmers[4] are at the root of Influenza A viruses' ability to mutate into deadlier forms is not necessarily accurate either. In 2013, journalist Laurie Garrett openly speculated that an incident involving hundreds of dead pigs found floating in a local river near Shanghai weeks earlier was somehow connected to the emergence of H7N9 (2013). After testing, no evidence that pigs were ever infected with the novel H7N9 subtype was found. Yet despite the emergence of H1N1 in Mexico in 2009, and mounting evidence that novel influenza strains can originate anywhere that wild birds, domesticated birds, swine, and humans are in close contact, China remains the principal site for global influenza surveillance. Recent models, based in part on data collected through routine surveillance in China, highlight China as a "hot spot" for viral recombinations—or future novel flu viruses (Fuller et. al. 2013).

In relationship to its geographical location and epidemiological history, then, the city of Hong Kong is seen not only as one of the epicenters of novel influenzas, but as a center of their potential global spread. Narratives that depict Hong Kong as a naturally diseased space underline how interconnected the biology of influenza is with its geography (and as we saw in the previous chapter, proximity to the "origin" of influenza viruses has had a positive impact on laboratories in the city). One cannot talk about biology without recourse to geography. Where influenza is said to originate matters to the creation of new narratives about who is well-placed to become a global flu expert and where the best research centers for influenza are located. Hong Kong has taken its stigmatized reputation as the source of global influenza to its logical and empowering conclusion; if someone wants to understand the virus, then she must do research in the city.

This rhetorical transformation of Hong Kong from a disease source into a resource is perhaps best understood in relationship to its postcolonial legacies. As will be explored in more depth below, Hong Kong is in a contiguous relationship to its colonial past. Being repatriated has not altered the sense of historical time and place that pervades the territory in the present. Not only is Hong Kong habitually conceptualized as being in between

East and West, but its present is often discursively cast as being somehow in between the colony's past and the global city's future. Viewed through the dual lenses of its postcoloniality and its "Chineseness," then, Hong Kong is always, to use political scholar Jean-François Bayart's phrasing, in "an interaction between the past, the present, and a projected future, but also an interaction between social actors or between societies" (2005, 137). The city's interstitial positioning vis-à-vis geography, time, and culture is a result of its imbrication in the process and practices of globalization itself. Indeed, and as anthropologist Johannes Fabian argues (1983), global modernity itself rests upon the creation of cultural differences through spatial and temporal distances. This type of postcolonial temporality—or looping back and forth in time and space between being a former British colony and a Chinese city—allows scientists working in the city to craft and enact unique local public health policies that, in turn, have had ripple effects within the global health community.[5] One might effectively even argue, then, that the postcolonial continues to "infect" the global. Nowhere has this infection been more visible than in relationship to the issue of quarantine.

Throughout the 2009 pandemic, I became intrigued by the ways in which Hong Kong public health officials talked about and defended their early response to H1N1—above all their decision to implement quarantine after the first case was discovered there in May. The reigning response to influenza pandemics in Western nations is mitigation (social distancing, hand-washing, and prophylaxis with antiviral medications) along with the development of vaccines. Indeed, mitigation is the universal strategy officially recommended by the WHO. In China, however, the national pandemic plan includes containment measures (quarantine, border screening, contact tracing, and school closures) *in addition to* mitigation tactics and national vaccine development. Containment, according to Chinese officials, "buys time" to prepare for pandemic response in developing countries that do not have resources or medical stockpiles akin to those of the United States or other Western nations. As a Special Administrative Region (SAR), Hong Kong is free to direct its own pandemic response and choose its actions in relationship to its own context and needs. Hong Kong's experience during the 2009 H1N1 pandemic can thus be seen as not only indicative of its interstitial position between worlds, but performative of it.

In what follows, I explore how Hong Kong's particular geography and history relate to its response actions in May 2009. Hong Kong's decision to quarantine is "good to think with" and from. Following Cori Hayden's examination of the "representational capacities of knowledge" (2003, 345), I use the example of quarantine to examine how epidemiological knowledge in Hong Kong is asked to represent either a "Chinese" or a "Western" standpoint. Debates over the effectiveness of quarantine help to delineate how geography, history, and culture matter not only to the practice of epidemiology, but increasingly to the formation of global expertise.

The Beginnings of Postcolonial-Global Public Health

Living in Hong Kong, one almost gets used to the idea of infection. Sporadic outbreaks of H5N1 in the live bird markets; the specter of SARS whenever someone with an acute, unexplained upper respiratory tract infection is hospitalized; the occasional case of Japanese encephalitis; thick, humid air that feels pregnant with microbes; the soundless, nearly invisible mosquitos ubiquitous in the lush, dense patches of forest that cover the territory. Contagions seem to originate both from within and from without, as seasonal outbreaks or strange events, but with a regularity that can induce lethargy instead of sharp anxiety.

In part, this infectious disease fatigue is an effect of living in a city that is conceptualized as one of the homes of influenza. In part, it is a symptom of living in a globalized world—in a city that is complexly interconnected to every other city on the planet. Infectious diseases can come, quite literally, from anywhere. Conceptualizations of infectious disease, on the other hand, have a long history of being associated with notions of the "Other," with the foreign, and as originating from the colony itself (Anderson 2006, Arnold 1993, Brandt 1987, Briggs and Mantini-Briggs 2003, Douglas 1966, Farmer 2006, Gilman 1988, Martin 1994, Wald 2008). Tracing the history of imperialism, Hardt and Negri argue that disease has historically been schematized as "a sign of physical and moral corruption, a sign of a lack of civilization." Actual contagion is indeed partly a product of globalizing forces, a result of the international flow of goods, people, and capital; imagined contagion, or fear of "universal contagion," is globalization's dark underbelly. (Hardt and Negri 2000, 135, 136.) Narratives about disease have always highlighted larger societal concerns about the transgression of boundaries, contact with "others," and miscegenation (Wald 2008). Yet this fear of contagion has also been wildly productive in terms of advancement in the biosciences; the connection between colonization and the development of improved systems of public health has been well explored (Porter 1999, Rosen 1958, Watts 1997). Global expansion created a need for better medicine. Colonies such as Hong Kong were the prima facie driving force for the first instantiations of global health systems.

From the very beginning of its British colonization, Hong Kong was seen as a reservoir—or pit—of disease. The island's so-called naturally disease-prone environment—its year-round humidity and swampy, tropical marshland—was conceptualized as an immense problem for its colonizers. The opening sentence of the Hong Kong Museum of Medical Sciences Society's account of the history of infectious disease in Hong Kong is a quote taken directly from a travelogue published in 1849. It reflects its British author's opinion, based upon years of extensive travel throughout the Middle Kingdom, that Hong Kong was unconditionally "the most unhealthy spot in China." Most troublesome to the Brits were a collection of diseases generically labeled as "Hongkong fever." (Ho 2006a, 17, 19.) Assumed to refer primarily to malaria, Hongkong fever killed troops by the hundreds. Historian John M. Carroll notes that in just one scant month, May 1843, the British lost nearly a quarter of their troops to malaria. Hongkong fever was so serious and so rife throughout the mid-nineteenth century that "a popular song in London music halls rang 'You may go to Hong Kong for me.'" (Carroll 2007, 19, 20.) The new port's reputation as a diseased space, it seemed, preceded it.

A series of similarly deadly outbreaks convinced the British government to take pains to stamp out infectious disease in the colony. Hospitals were built and Western medical authorities were brought in to cope with the seemingly never-ending series of infectious diseases—each wave of which threatened to overwhelm Hong Kong's British and Chinese inhabitants and destroy its bustling economy. And although Hong Kong was certainly no stranger to disease, it was ultimately a particularly fatal outbreak of plague that would become the catalyst for the establishment of what would evolve into Hong Kong's first modern scientific research center: the Bacteriological Institute.

In 1894, an outbreak of plague in the Western District of Hong Kong Island provided bacteriologists trained in the methods of Pasteur and

Koch with a unique opportunity to investigate whether or not a particular disease agent was the definitive cause of the plague. Merely a decade had elapsed since Koch's discovery of the tuberculosis bacillus, and germ theory remained a relatively new science. Bacteriologists were eager to prove the effectiveness of their skills and bolster their nascent scientific field. Particularly high mortality rates in the active trade port attracted the interest of the entire international scientific community. Acting on the authority of the British government, Japan sent a team of scientists to Hong Kong to investigate the outbreak. At the same time, a French national working for the newly established Pasteur Institute in Vietnam, Alexandre Yersin, heard about the outbreak and traveled to Hong Kong with support from the French government, but without official consent from the British authorities. The resulting scientific race to isolate the plague bacillus began almost immediately. Although the Japanese team technically won, credit for the discovery of the bacillus ultimately went to Yersin, whose scientific description was deemed more complete and accurate than that of his Japanese rivals.

Within this early narrative of disease research in Hong Kong can be observed the outlines of a developing friction between "Eastern" and "Western" scientific methods and expertise. Perhaps unsurprisingly, then, the plague outbreak also highlighted brewing tensions between British and Chinese residents. The high virulence and sheer persistence of the plague were blamed on the unsanitary conditions of the Chinese living quarters in Tai Ping Shan. Western and traditional Chinese medicine were pitted against each other in attempts to exterminate the disease (Ho 2006a, 31). Since the British authorities were ostensibly able to control the plague, if not to eradicate it outright, the outbreak can be viewed as the entry point that allowed Western medicine to gain a foothold among the Chinese in Hong Kong.[6] Following plague in 1894, British authorities enforced the increased implementation of Western standards of medicine in Chinese hospitals and insisted that English become a routine part of Chinese education (Carroll 2007).

Plague in Hong Kong lasted for the next thirty years and caused over twenty thousand deaths. A booklet detailing the 1894 outbreak, for sale at the Medical Museum in commemoration of the hundredth anniversary of the founding of Hong Kong's Bacteriological Institute, details how persistent outbreaks of plague disrupted Hong Kong's economy (Ho 2006b, 17).

As a result, the disease became an issue of critical importance for the British government. As a port, Hong Kong was an integral part of the overall British economy; plague threatened to close the port to traffic and halt the lucrative flow of goods. To prevent this type of disruption, the governor of Hong Kong determined that the colony needed "a laboratory for original research" on disease. The renowned scientist Patrick Manson (1844–1922), considered by many medical historians to be the father of tropical medicine, became an early and vocal promoter of the development of "first rate clinical and research work in medicine and public health" in Hong Kong. According to Ho's account, Manson was desirous that Hong Kong become a "Centre for Science for the whole of China and not just a centre for merchandise." (Ho 2006b, 18, 20.) Manson managed to convince William Hunter, a brilliant bacteriologist working in London, that Hong Kong held out a multitude of unique research opportunities. Hunter agreed to relocate to the colony to set up the Bacteriological Institute.

After years of costly expenditures and shipments of pricey equipment from Europe, the Bacteriological Institute officially opened in 1906. The institute was erected at the center of Tai Ping Shan—the poor, Chinese section of the city that had been blamed for the start of the plague and subsequently razed in an effort to halt the spread of the disease. The decision to build the new institute at the site of the plague's alleged origin point was emblematic; a symbol of Western scientific medicine constructed literally at the center of Hong Kong's most diseased space.

A solid, colonial-style building, the former Bacteriological Institute (now the Medical Museum) is imposing. Its structure—a red brick façade towering three floors above street level—has both an institutional and a homelike quality to it. Inside, high ceilings and large windows let in copious amounts of light and create the illusion of an airy and healthy enclosure for scientific investigation. At its center is a dumb waiter used to hoist materials from the basement—where the autopsy rooms and morgue were located—to the bright and spacious second and third floors—the location of the building's largest working laboratory.

Despite having a state-of-the-art research laboratory, the institute's main tasks remained plague surveillance and vaccine production. Regular duties left scientists with little leftover time for conducting original scientific research. However, the institute's additional role as the city's mortuary eventually led Dr. Hunter to the realization that the bodies of deceased

Hong Kongers[7] might provide him with a "wide range of disease conditions" for scientific investigation. The city's morgue concealed a "rare research potential" (Ho 2006b, 50). Thus, the morgue turned the city into a disease resource for Hunter.

With tissue samples obtained from the mortuary, Hunter created a pathology museum, one eventually used to train Chinese medical students at the University of Hong Kong. An early researcher at the Institute mused that "'If the newcomer is a Pathologist, he will at once be struck by the abundance of material to be found in the Public Mortuary daily. . . . The opportunities for original research are practically unlimited.'" (Ho 2006b, 59, 63.) Here, Hong Kong is rhetorically crafted as a rich natural resource for the mining of disease agents. Working at the Bacteriological Institute provided scientists with material for further scientific discovery. New and interesting pathogens awaited those scientists bold enough to relocate to the British colony to conduct research. The entire island, then, becomes envisioned as a type of "living laboratory" for international research on infectious disease.

At the end of the museum's booklet, author Faith Ho argues that the Bacteriological Institute is the precursor of Hong Kong's renowned Centre for Health Protection (CHP). The institute had "been brought into existence in response to the plague outbreak, in the same way that the latter was brought about in response to the SARS outbreak" (Ho 2006b, 86). The parallel drawn here between institutes, time periods, and the changing status of Western medicine and public health is striking. In this account, the location of scientific buildings is put in historical and geographic relationship to the quality of research conducted within them. If geography matters to biology, then the biological past becomes a way to explain the location of research centers. The Chinese phrase 古为今用 (*gǔ wéi jīn yòng*)—translated as "making the past serve the present"—illuminates how narratives about Hong Kong's diseased past are being reshaped to serve the needs of those working in global public health in the city today.

古为今用: The Colonial Past in the Global Present

In 2008, the University of Hong Kong Art Museum curated an exhibition for the anniversary of the establishment of the HKU-Pasteur Research

Center—internationally recognized as one of the premier research laboratories not only in the SAR, but in all of Southeast Asia. Yersin's discovery of the plague bacillus in Hong Kong in 1894 was on prominent display. At the middle of the main exhibit hall stood a straw hut, a full-size replica of Yersin's original makeshift research laboratory, complete with a lifesize cutout of Yersin that invited the museum goer to quite literally measure herself against the leading figure of Hong Kong's epidemiological past. Walking around the exhibit, it became clear to me that the plague story is central not only to the history of medical science in Hong Kong, but to the Pasteur Institute's story of its historical collaboration with Hong Kong scientists. In the Art Museum's retelling of the Yersin story, continuity with the present moment takes center stage; the epidemic past is being made to serve the public health present.

I interpret the comingling of Yersin's historical discovery with the work done in the twenty-first century on SARS and influenza at the Pasteur Institute as a visual and palpable linkage between Hong Kong's past and present. The past—as symbolized by Yersin's work on the plague—was meant to speak for the present work being done by the HKU-Pasteur Institute. The city's experience with plague is thereby placed in historical context *as part of* Hong Kong's recent experience with SARS and avian influenza. The colonial past is—quite literally—connected to the present and future of microbiology in Asia's global city.

In the exhibition catalog, the curator made these linkages even more obvious, writing that "Yersin's significance in the development of public health provisions in Hong Kong also makes him a fitting introduction to the science of virology, its history and its continuing importance today. In this exhibition, we hope that by understanding how Hong Kong has been affected by infectious diseases in the past, and through the work of Yersin, that visitors might better appreciate the challenges that virologists face today, such as dengue fever, avian influenza, and SARS" (University of Hong Kong 2008, 17). In many ways, the story as retold through both the museum display and the catalogue is a hero's tale. Yersin is portrayed as scientist, adventurer, and victor over his "natural" foes—the plague bacilli. The competition between Yersin and the Japanese team is highlighted, with Yersin prevailing. The story of the discovery of the plague bacillus is recounted through beautiful pictorials of Yersin's experiences in Southeast Asia and in Hong Kong, along with displays of various notebooks and artifacts such as old microscopes and science kits. Samples extracted from Hong Kong corpses, which Yersin did not technically have permission to obtain, were taken back to Paris and used to develop a serum for plague. That serum then traveled back to Hong Kong as a product of Parisian scientific expertise and technological know-how. Hong Kong and Paris are fused here—in the past as in the present—through the circulation of knowledge and objects, as well as through the collaborative practice of international disease research.

Of particular interest in the Art Museum's exhibit catalogue is a two-page spread near its end that shows the evolution of scientific research on infectious disease. Foregrounded on the left-hand page are a collection of old bottles, an old microscope, and an open book. The book is obviously very old, hand-bound in leather, and opened to a page that shows both text and a colorful illustration. The book is the visual connection between the past and the present. Directly above the text of the book on the right-hand side of the page, a researcher clad in a modern biosecurity suit is shown pipetting something into a small test tube. Next to him, and as opposed to the ancient, outdated microscope on the left-hand side of the page, a modern centrifuge. This pictorial montage is a prelude to the final pages of the brochure, which juxtapose the historical story of plague in Hong Kong with its effect on modern disease research, surveillance, and prevention. The brochure ends with a claim that "The 'continued presence' of plague in Hong Kong at the turn of the 20th century turned it into a place vigilant of, and responsive to, diseases and their life-threatening potential. The plague of 1894, and Alexandre Yersin's discovery of the plague bacillus that bears his name, made medical history, and located Hong Kong as an important gatekeeper in the prevention of worldwide epidemics" (University of Hong Kong 2008, 59). This rhetorical stance turns Hong Kong from a *colonial diseased space* into a *global disease source* and one of the vigilant protectors of global health. But here the concept of "source" is not viewed in relationship to stigmatization. Rather, Hong Kong's long history of being a passive site of contagion is turned into a positive attribute that reflects its commitment to becoming a responsible and active partner in global health. The city is thus reconceptualized as an abundant resource, the site of the raw material needed for advancing science. Hong Kong's present-day scientists and public health workers here are cast as active participants in the "global fight" against infectious disease, and Hong Kongers are thereby rhetorically transformed from passive "colonial subjects" into active and responsible "global citizens."

When I visited the former Bacteriological Institute in the spring of 2010, the main exhibition was a detailed history of Hong Kong's more recent (and triumphant) experience with SARS. The exhibit materials stressed the success of Hong Kong's public health system and, in an echo of Yersin's story of over a hundred years before, lionized the top virologists who discovered the SARS coronavirus. Except that unlike in 1894, these microbiologists were "native" to Asia, hailing from Sri Lanka and Hong Kong. The city's display of pride in its homegrown infectious disease research and surveillance capacity, while not unfounded, is an interesting counterpoint to its historical legacy as a diseased space. In the ensuing century, Hong Kong has evidently learned to utilize its conceptualization as a place rife with disease to its own distinct advantage.

Disease, one might argue, is one of Hong Kong's natural resources. Access to its viral and bacterial samples guarantees Hong Kong scientists a permanent position in developing global disease networks. At the same time, and not unrelatedly, access to those samples grants local researchers and scientists an unparalleled opportunity for innovation and progress. Hong Kong's past as a disease *source* is now working to its advantage as a disease *resource* for scientific research. The past—including the Bacteriological Institute—has been incorporated into a newer narrative that both undergirded the development of the Centre for Health Protection and is used to secure Hong Kong's position as a global leader of future developments in epidemiological science. In a city that prides itself on its modernity, what might the preservation of the old Bacteriological Institute—and its eventual transformation into the Hong Kong Medical Museum—tell us about Hong Kong's unfolding relationship to its past and present as a diseased space?

Historian John M. Carroll suggests that such preservation projects "promote a sense of Hong Kong localness and belonging within a larger sense of Chinese nationalism" (2007, 237). Hong Kong scholar Ackbar Abbas, writing about Hong Kong's relationship to the preservation of its colonial past, argues that "The preservation of old buildings gives us history in site, but it also means keeping history in sight" (1997, 66). Looking at the Bacteriological Institute through this lens, the building is an example of Hong Kong's unique history. It is particular only to Hong Kong, imbued with the city's colonial past as an important trade hub and center of British colonial rule. It encapsulates and makes real Hong Kong's postcoloniality in the present moment. The newly-built Centre for Health Protection, the modern equivalent of the Bacteriological Institute, is an example of what Abbas might term a "placeless" facility (1997, 83). Unlike the institute, the CHP is a large, nondescript, modern-industrial building that one might find in any city. The CHP is thus representative of Hong Kong's current role in global public health; it is an interchangeable part in the larger network. The two buildings are linked through time and space and, as a result, their meanings are kept in constant interplay. Together, they construct Hong Kong as a natural disease resource and a center for cutting-edge research. Thus the Bacteriological Institute acts as a kind of placeholder for the colonial history of Hong Kong as a source of disease. The building's careful preservation, then, becomes integral to the emergent story that the Hong Kong medical and scientific communities construct about their ability to do important infectious disease research in the city today.

What is interesting about historical accounts of plague, as written by Ho and embodied in the former Bacteriological Institute itself, is that Hong Kong is highlighted not only as a site for the discovery of disease or as an "incubator" for tropical disease, but as having played an integral role in the development of present-day global public health. The postcolonial here is transformed into the global. As "teaching texts," the museum booklet and exhibits produce the history of microbiology and epidemiology in Hong Kong, casting the city not as a passive site for research, but as a contributor "to the knowledge of the disease, its cause, its control and prevention" (Ho 2006a, 36). Hong Kong is reconceptualized as the source of and contributor to knowledge about infectious diseases—avian influenza and SARS being given particular emphasis near the end of Ho's historical account. In closing, Ho writes that "Hong Kong is therefore rightly part of the global scientific community and can be proud of the fact that it now participates in it on an equal footing with others in the best medical centers of the world's developed countries. *We can see how this has changed over the years from plague to SARS*" (2006a, 73).

The museum booklet thus takes pains to reappropriate the Bacteriological Institute, originally British, as part of Hong Kong's singular legacy. Ho argues: "Let us give back a little recognition to this unsung hero, the 'Silent Protector,' the place where much of the early work on health protection was carried out, and learn to appreciate and treasure this little corner of our Hong Kong heritage" (Ho 2006b, 8). The booklet itself poses and answers the question of why Hong Kongers should still care about such a history. Dr. Lo Wing-Lok argues in the booklet's introduction that "When we are almost fully consumed by the cares of the present and by the uncertainties of the future, why do we need to trouble ourselves with the past? My answer to that is our present was very much shaped by the past and our present will to a large extent determine our future" (Ho 2006b, 7). The colonial *past*, as depicted and retold through these texts and museum displays, is very much *present*. It is being called upon to do foundational work in the narrative that Hong Kong scripts about itself as a global research center and as an active, responsible partner in global public health. This narrative was then highlighted and underscored during the SARS outbreak in 2003.

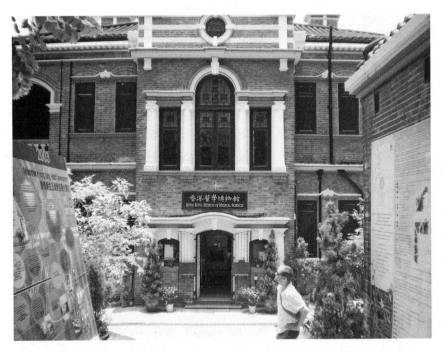

Figure 10. The former Bacteriological Institute. This is the front view of what is now the Museum of Medical Sciences in the summer of 2008. Visible on the left is part of the exhibit on the 2003 SARS outbreak.

Quarantine in Hong Kong, Part One—SARS

The 2003 SARS coronavirus outbreak initially began in late 2002 in Guangdong Province. By early 2003, Hong Kong's public health officials were on high alert for cases of atypical pneumonia inside the Special Administrative Region. As any local epidemiologist can attest, an outbreak of infectious disease in one location usually predicates an outbreak in its neighbor. Hong Kong is connected to Guangdong not just geographically and spatially, but economically and culturally. Outbreaks of infectious disease connect Hong Kong to mainland China as readily as the region's long history of cross-border migration and trade. So in late February 2003, when the first SARS patient (a doctor who had previously treated SARS patients in Guangzhou, the capital of Guangdong Province) was discovered in Hong Kong, it did not exactly come as a huge surprise. What did surprise Hong Kong's public health experts was the overwhelming severity of the outbreak. By late March, large clusters of SARS infections at the Prince of Wales Hospital and the Amoy Gardens residential complex had necessitated the implementation of aggressive public health measures: quarantine, isolation, contact tracing, and border screening. By the time local public health officials had wrestled the novel virus into abeyance, over 1,700 Hong Kong citizens had been directly affected by the disease. Public health experts traced the index patient in Hong Kong to 156 contacts, some of whom had spread SARS to seven different countries. By the end of the global outbreak in July 2003, over 8,000 cases of SARS had been reported to the WHO with 775 deaths—the overwhelming majority in Hong Kong (299 fatalities) and mainland China (349 fatalities). Hong Kong's quick response would not only be praised by the international public health community[8] for helping to halt a global epidemic, but held up as a shining example of effective public health response to infectious disease in the twenty-first century. Thus the outbreak of SARS had two major and interlocking effects on Hong Kong: it enriched the city's reputation as a vigilant and responsible partner in global health at the same time that it highlighted and deepened Hong Kong's increasingly complex relationship with mainland China.

Throughout 2003, media coverage of SARS had depicted Hong Kong as a Chinese and diseased city. In a book on the aftermath of the crisis, former Hong Kong Legislative Council member Christine Loh recounts that Hong Kong, the New Territories, and Guangdong Province were collectively described by the international community as "a natural Petri dish for pathogens" and as "China's Petri Dish to the World." International media portrayed Hong Kong during SARS as a "death city"; the preventative face mask donned by its citizens quickly became the ubiquitous media symbol that (re)constructed Hong Kong as a diseased space. Yet Loh reminds us that the experience of SARS also provided Hong Kong with an opportunity to see itself as a capable and successful scientific and epidemiological community. Loh argues that "half of all scientific publications related to SARS" were published by local experts, and that Hong Kong microbiologists in particular "had received international attention." (Loh 2004, 7, 198, 196, 197, 223.) Indeed, the two University of Hong Kong microbiologists who discovered the SARS coronavirus were subsequently held up as paragons of the global public health community. Post-SARS, Hong Kong—and, by extension, China as a whole—had cemented its vital role in emergent global public health networks.

And yet if SARS had highlighted the city's increasingly close relationship with the Chinese mainland, then it had also reinstantiated much older

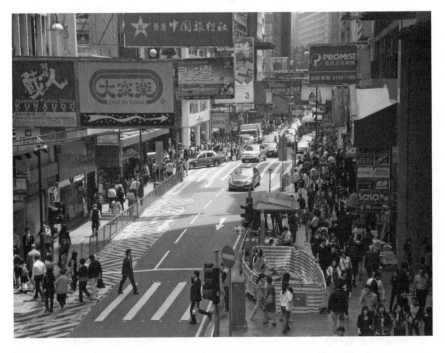

Figure 11. A typical working-day view in Central District, Hong Kong.

debates about Hong Kong's relative Chinese- or British-ness. In effect, the SARS crisis exposed Hong Kong's spatial location and historical positioning between mainland China and the rest of the world. The territory's former status as a British colony and its continued relationships with the UK and the United States (what I will refer to throughout the remainder of this chapter as "the West") were reexamined through larger international discussions about its actions during SARS. Post-SARS, Hong Kong was made to simultaneously stand in for "Western" and "Chinese" approaches to the practice of public health. Throughout the crisis in 2003, Hong Kong's decisions had been compared to those of the mainland partially in order to, as it were, prove the effectiveness of Western or universal methods of infectious disease response. Hong Kong was largely seen as a modern and already globalized city. As a former British colony that retained traces of both a Western public health approach and a hybridized political structure, the city was praised by the WHO for its quick and appropriate response to the crisis: its quarantining of hotel guests and residents of the Amoy Gardens complex, its transparency throughout the outbreak, and its key role in identifying and helping to halt the spread of the novel SARS coronavirus. China's initial reaction to the crisis, on the other hand, had been castigated by the WHO and the international public health community as less than exemplary. In comparison to Hong Kong, the mainland's faults were seen as many: early reports on the outbreak had not been made transparent in a timely manner;[9] the Chinese national disease surveillance system had also been slow to react, allowing the crisis to deepen; and Chinese authorities were seen as largely bungling the early response by controlling access to both information and patients, thus worsening an already serious situation. Thus, China, with its authoritarian political structure and ineffective or "backward" public health infrastructure, was (for the most part accurately) accused of directly and indirectly enabling the spread of SARS. Significantly, however, once the crisis had gone public in Hong Kong, the Chinese Communist Party quickly reversed its actions on the mainland. In April, the Chinese government mobilized its substantial public health resources, quarantining thousands of patients and school children, canceling the national week-long May 1 holiday (when millions of Chinese travel to visit family), and implementing effective containment measures in hospitals in order to control the outbreak's further spread. By the end of May, China had stopped SARS—in part by imitating Hong Kong's practices and adapting them to the mainland. Events in 2003 highlighted the congruities and differences between the city and the mainland, but the combined resultant "Chinese-style intervention was extolled as a means of controlling future epidemics" (Kleinman and Watson 2006, 4–5). By the end of the crisis, then, Hong Kong as a global Chinese city had been positioned as a resource and model for both China and the West.

After the SARS crisis, Hong Kong experts continued to collaborate with their mainland counterparts, even if the relationship was sometimes strained. Scientist and scholar Alexis Lau notes that during the SARS crisis few in Hong Kong "took the reports from across the border seriously, because of a lack of trust either in China's capacity in disease control and prevention or in the accuracy of data" (2004, 86). In point of fact, however, SARS was a watershed moment for cross-border cooperation in public health. As a policy expert noted, "SARS revealed weaknesses in the 'one country, two systems' framework that are now leading to changes in the relationship between Hong Kong and its immediate hinterlands in the Pearl River Delta and Guangdong Province" (DeGolyer 2004, 137). In other words, the SARS virus acted as a physical and conceptual link that helped to integrate Hong Kong back into mainland China. An acute outbreak of infectious disease had done what years of economic cooperation had failed to do—it forced the former British colony to directly confront its past, present, and future relationship to mainland China.

Politician Christine Loh suggests that the outbreak of SARS was one of the first major impetuses for what would become a series of pioneering cross-border agreements, with both Hong Kong and Guangdong Province agreeing to share information on outbreaks more freely and to continue to foster better cooperation. Loh writes that "Hong Kong now sees itself more clearly as part of the neighborhood of Guangdong Province. Furthermore, it has also become more evident that Hong Kong is an integral part of China, although it functions as a Special Administrative Region." As current under secretary for the environment in Hong Kong, Loh links these agreements, themselves a result of the SARS crisis, to China's "drive for modernization," with Hong Kong conceptualized here as already modern. Continued integration is part of an "opportunity to create the model for new China." (Loh 2004, 157, 140, 160.) Here Hong Kong is regarded not only as part of China, but as integral to China's development and modernization in the twenty-first century. If throughout China's more recent history, Hong Kong had been cast as a proxy for China (Evans and Tam

1997, Hughes 1968, Lo 2005), then what Loh's comments highlight is how the city is being reconceptualized as a model for and as a representation of today's China. This reassertion of Hong Kong's position as a Chinese city is important not only in relationship to SARS, science, and public health, but to geopolitics on the grand scale. Hong Kong has become a weather vane to divine the direction of Chinese policies. Hong Kong here is the future of Chinese approaches to global health.

Hong Kong scholar Kwai-Cheung Lo argues that Hong Kong has always been a "crack in the edifice of Chineseness" that simultaneously "exaggerates and negates Chineseness" (2005, 4) on the global stage. For Lo, the effects of Hong Kong's colonial past are very much present in the positioning of Hong Kong as a modern Chinese city. He writes that

> To many foreign visitors, Hong Kong already appears to be a very "Chinese" city. It was used to exhibit Chineseness when the "real" China could not be accessed. In fact, the returned Hong Kong may serve as an exemplar of Chineseness not because the colonial city disassociated from Chinese culture in order to produce a Hong Kong identity, but because it has been producing and reshaping Chineseness since the early colonial era. For decades, Hong Kong's popular culture has succeeded in creating and perpetuating an abstract kind of Chinese nationalism and identity for a global audience. (2005, 3)

Hong Kong is thus an example of what Ackbar Abbas has termed a "post-culture," defined as "a culture that has developed in a situation where the available models of culture no longer work." Within this framework, Hong Kong is experienced as a series of instabilities (1997, 145) wherein binaries and boundaries break down. Anthropologist Tim Choy has argued against using too easy binarisms and concepts to describe Hong Kong, urging us instead to look at "how particularity comes to work as a mark of expertise" (2005, 6) in the territory. There is no such thing as Chinese or Western, or Chinese or Western science, or Chinese or Western epidemiology and public health.[10] There is only Hong Kong and its particular style of response to outbreaks of infectious diseases. Any knowledge produced in the city must be simultaneously universal and particular in order for it to be effective.

Indeed, scientists and epidemiologists working in Hong Kong are hyper-aware of their roles as both local and international scientists. In discussions about their work, Hong Kong researchers and epidemiologists regularly "code-switched" (Evans and Tam 1997, 5), or talked about themselves and the scientific product of their research as up to international or universal scientific standards on one hand, and as representative of the local situation on the other. One local researcher even bemoaned to me that "Unfortunately, Hong Kong is more British than the British. You know, the colonial roots . . . you just cannot unplug." Scientists and epidemiologists often described their work as relevant and important to the international scientific community at large, but also particular to the situation in Hong Kong. They located both themselves and their research in larger professional and personal networks. In interviews, they regularly discussed their developing relationship to their Chinese counterparts in Guangdong or Beijing, always noting how much better the situation was in 2010 than it had been in 2003 during SARS.

Despite declarations of an increasingly close working relationship between China and the SAR, scientists in Hong Kong often still expressed a lingering mistrust of their counterparts across the border—a leftover, if you will, from the region's experience with SARS. At issue was not just personal trust, but professional capacities. Local experts were also often self-reflective about the overt politics—and competition—associated with doing influenza research in the region. As one scientist articulated it to me, infectious diseases like influenza or SARS were "inevitably political." Hong Kong's interstitial role—as both Chinese and global, neither British nor Chinese—seemed to play a crucial role in how scientists and epidemiologists positioned themselves and their research within larger global networks. This interstitial positioning is an effect of not only Hong Kong's geographical location but its history as a colony and center for research on infectious disease.

Hong Kong signifies much more than just "Chineseness" or what might be conceptualized outside of Hong Kong as a particularly "Chinese" brand of practicing public health. The city, along with its local epidemiological expertise, is perhaps best viewed as a weather vane pointing the way toward a more complex, interconnected, future. Hong Kong's self-consciousness about its global and local position—and its limits—enable it "to link different subject positions into an overarching struggle" (Chen 2010, 99) to maintain its political autonomy and its unique status as a Special Administrative Region of China. Hong Kong, then, has clear implications for how we can think about things like global health, nationalism, and post-coloniality in the twenty-first century. Hong Kong simply does not fit comfortably inside any theory or system—be it postcolonial theory,[11] theories related to identity and nationalism, or the system of global public health. Or, as Kwai-Cheung Lo has argued, Hong Kong's Western-Chineseness underlies its unique position as the Switzerland of Asia—positioned as existing both "inside and outside of China"—thus making it representative of a "new understanding of Chineseness and its interplay with today's world" (2005, 2). Hong Kong's relationships to its own epidemiological past, to mainland China, and to the larger international public health community, its postcolonial temporality and interstitial positioning, have all allowed it to retain a certain flexibility in choosing its own course of action. That flexibility, in turn, was the foundational basis for the adaptability of its response during the earliest weeks of the 2009 H1N1 pandemic.

Quarantine in Hong Kong, Part Two—H1N1

Living in a "space of flow" (Castells 2010) for finance, goods, and people, Hong Kongers know better than anyone else that in a globalized world, infectious diseases travel through the nodes of the network with lightning speed; viruses don't usually linger in one area for long. So when public health officials and scientists in Hong Kong heard about the late seasonal H1N1 outbreak in Mexico in March–April 2009,[12] they knew with absolute certainty that it would travel—and travel fast. The question became not "if" Hong Kong should prepare for an outbreak of H1N1, but "how long" the city might have to activate its emergency response systems and how best to prepare.

On May 1, 2009, the first case of H1N1 was detected in Hong Kong. A twenty-five-year-old Mexican citizen traveling to Hong Kong from Shanghai came down with a fever and was immediately placed in isolation at Princess Margaret Hospital. The hotel where the infected man had been staying—located in the densely populated Wanchai District on Hong Kong Island—was placed in quarantine for the following seven days. In total, approximately three hundred people were quarantined, including hotel guests, staff, and any airline passengers sitting within five rows of the index patient. Following the detection of the first case of H1N1, authorities in Beijing decided to cancel all direct flights from Mexico to China, an act that initiated a minor and public diplomatic scuffle between the two nations. Hong Kong (and China) defended its actions in terms of prior experiences with SARS, local epidemiological studies and expertise, and the city's geographic location. The heavily contextual decision to quarantine was thus located in relationship to Hong Kong's postcolonial temporality as both a SARS survivor, a unique place, and part of the larger global public health network.

Subsequent debates about the effectiveness of quarantine for influenza were ultimately part of larger debates about the construction of expertise in global public health. I often found myself puzzling about the problem of quarantine as it was couched by non–Hong Kongers, as a particularly Chinese reaction to outbreaks of infectious disease. How and why had a brief quarantine in Hong Kong instantiated a larger deliberation about the effectiveness of different public health responses? What was local knowledge about the effectiveness of quarantine being asked to do or to represent in the construction of universal knowledge about how best to cope with influenza pandemics? It seemed to me that discussions about quarantine were part of the negotiation of universally applicable "best practices" for influenza pandemics and about whose voices would shape that knowledge.

As a member of the WHO Influenza Network and the Global Influenza Surveillance Network, and in relationship to the city's past successes with containing outbreaks, one might predict that Hong Kong's choice to quarantine during the 2009 H1N1 pandemic would meet with the same international approval as its decision to quarantine during SARS in 2003. Instead, the response was perceived outside of China as an overreaction. Most public health professionals working in the United States and Europe view quarantine as a largely worthless measure to take against influenza. Notoriously difficult to contain, flu is principally dealt with in Western nations through the mitigation efforts mentioned earlier. But in Hong Kong and China, the thinking has always been slightly different. As Hong Kongers repeatedly explained to me, the SAR is unique in that it is a small and densely populated area. As such, it has resources and systems in place to quarantine effectively, as well as a social system prepared to cope with short- and long-term school closures. What's more, as I was continually reminded, the local populace expected quarantine, almost demanded it. In sum, Hong Kong's experts assert that containment measures like quarantine work in Hong Kong and China when they wouldn't work anywhere else.

Outside of Hong Kong and China, containment measures against the 2009 H1N1 virus were often identified as being based on "questionable" or scant scientific data regarding their overall effectiveness. I was repeatedly assured off the record that Hong Kong's quarantine and school closure measures were simply political or cultural, that there was little or no empirical evidence to suggest that quarantine was effective against the importation of influenza. From a Western perspective, then, Hong Kong quarantined because it could, because China did, and/or because it had a different "culture."

Quarantine is, and has always been, a tricky subject—economically, politically, and socially. It has never been seen as an entirely neutral act. As historian Sheldon Watts has shown, even during the height of the plague years in Europe, quarantine was often met with overt public hostility. Ordinary citizens, though frightened by a severe outbreak for the first week, quickly "grew accustomed to its depredations and, when left alone, attempted to go about their ordinary affairs" (Watts 1997, 18). Quarantine, then as now, disrupts the routine traffic of goods and people; outbreaks of plague have always occasioned official intrusions into the daily practices of entire populaces; and quarantine is thus often understood as an aggressive or excessively authoritative action. Quarantine policy is a reflection of "the levels to which a state chooses to intervene in the activities of its citizens, and it plays an important role in the types of regulations that govern the movement of foreign persons or goods across its borders" (Maglen 2003, 2873). Historically, quarantine was always as much a political tool between states as it was a method of preventing contagion. As Watts depicts again and again in his work on the political and social effects of infectious diseases throughout the centuries, outbreaks were indeed perfect opportunities for ruling authorities to intervene in the daily affairs of the public, creating what Watts calls an "Ideology of Order" (1997, 16). Outbreaks of disease are always conceptualized as localized, but also universal afflictions. They occur in a specific place—thus acquiring an "origin" or an unofficial nomenclature (such as Spanish flu)—but are also seen as generalized threats to global public health. Thus authorities have historically been able to justify quarantine in a locality by recourse to the language of protecting universal or global health. As Foucault points out, quarantine is a "limit case," an extreme form of "authoritarian medicalization" (1984, 275). Quarantine is as much about social control and the policing of the social body as it is about the "idea of the pathogenic city" (Foucault 1984, 282).

Events like quarantine in Hong Kong, then, are never "just" about quarantine or "just" about Hong Kong. Kwai-Cheung Lo argues that "The Hong Kong issue, when put in the context of international politics, is never confined to a local or national problem but is conceived in terms of a 'global design' for the remaking of the power hierarchy in the world" (2005, 13). As a former British colony, Hong Kong's recent decision to quarantine is partially conceptualized by non–Hong Kongers as a manifestation of its growing political alignment with China. Hong Kong's actions during the 2009 pandemic matter, then, partially because they are viewed as enactments of politics by other means. If the ability and willingness to quarantine is often couched as a direct reflection of a nation's larger political policies and ideologies, such as those concerning the control of immigration and trade (Maglen 2003), then we might argue that quarantine in Hong Kong is seen as being representative of Chinese authoritarianism itself.

What follows is an amalgamation of several interviews I conducted in April 2010 with top-ranking epidemiologists in Hong Kong. Some were native to Hong Kong and obtained extensive Western training in their field (in either the UK, the United States, or Australia). Some were British expats who had worked in Hong Kong for years, sometimes decades. Almost everyone had vast experience collaborating with their counterparts in mainland China and in the United States. As such, they were positioned as natural "translators" of epidemiological science, adept at packaging Western techniques and ideas for application both in the SAR and in Guangdong Province. Literally and metaphorically, then, they were seen as being able to speak multiple languages, often all at once. Their explanations for quarantine symbolize the cultural politics at stake in the recent public health responses to the 2009 H1N1 pandemic. More than this, however, they highlight the tensions inherent in Hong Kong's interstitial position between two overlapping, yet distinct, "cultures" of public health: China and the United States. Hong Kong's *cultural context*—as a SARS survivor, a Chinese SAR, and a global city—became preeminent in its rationale for its response to the 2009 pandemic.

Juxtaposed against these local viewpoints are comments from top epidemiologists working outside of China—reactions to Hong Kong's and China's decisions to quarantine collected in the United States at various times throughout the summer and fall of 2009. The resultant reconstructed "dialogue" about the effectiveness of quarantine below reveals an overtly Western concern about the correct Chinese translation or interpretation of scientific data. In its official decision to quarantine, Hong Kong appears to identify as "Chinese" rather than as "universal" in its logic. Hong Kong's decision can thus be read two ways: as symbolic of geopolitics in the twenty-first century and as part of the enactment of Hong Kong's viral expertise.

Slowing Down a Pandemic: Quarantine from Hong Kong's Perspective

From Hong Kong's and China's vantage point, quarantine is seen as a particularly effective tactic for slowing down the spread of the influenza virus during the earliest stages of a pandemic. Hong Kong's experts concurred with their US and European colleagues that importation of influenza cannot be stopped through containment. What the two sides disagreed on was whether containment was an effective strategy for slowing down the virus's spread, buying time to prepare for a severe outbreak if necessary. As many Hong Kong epidemiologists reminded me, information on the severity of the novel H1N1 was still inconclusive on May 1, when the first case was discovered in the SAR. The decision to quarantine was made based on several factors and was not an easy one for authorities to make; it was often described to me as a hedged bet, one that would have paid off if the outbreak had been worse than it was.

As Thomas Tsang, then controller of the Centre for Health Protection, described the situation to me:

> It was not an easy decision, actually, because you're talking about quarantining three hundred–plus people for a seven-day period. But we thought that we had to do this. Because it was the first case in Hong Kong and we were very worried that this would be a highly lethal infection, according to the initial reports that came out of Mexico. And with the experience of SARS, particularly since SARS actually happened in a hotel in the first place in Hong Kong, we thought that history was repeating itself. . . .

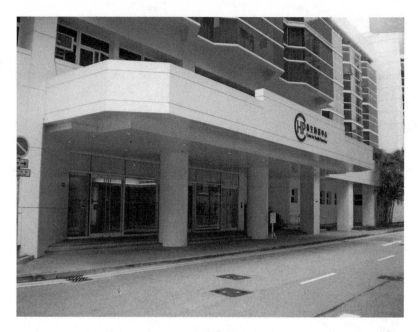

Figure 12. The Centre for Health Protection, Kowloon.

I think from the eyes of the American people, they would have thought that this would be a drastic action, right? Oh, this is just flu. Why all the fuss about quarantining a whole hotel, three hundred people for seven days? But I think Hong Kong, because we went through SARS—it was a very painful experience, OK? So both from a public health angle and from a political angle, I think, by and large, the local people supported this action.

Two lines of reasoning begin to emerge here. First, the choice to quarantine—as a decision that was framed as being particularly difficult to make—is predicated on a relationship to the past. Hong Kong's recent experience with SARS, then, is quite literally present during the 2009 outbreak of H1N1, and forms part of the logic or rationale for quarantine. Second, the justification for quarantine in Hong Kong is self-reflexively located in opposition to the United States' decision not to attempt to contain the virus. Hong Kong's action is partially conceptualized through the gaze of other experts—in this case, experts working inside the United States. For his part, Dr. Tsang is cognizant here of being representative of both Hong Kong's point of view and a global epidemiological authority.

Gabriel Leung, then under secretary at the Food and Health Bureau, echoed the rationale of his colleague Dr. Tsang. As one of the top public health officials during the outbreak, he offered the following explanation of Hong Kong's decision to use containment measures against the 2009 H1N1 virus:

> Well, we have never really stopped border screening in terms of thermal screening, infrared thermal screening. We've never stopped since SARS. We also in particular targeted flights from North America at the very beginning. And I think that's been effective, and essential, at the earliest stages. The WHO phase four is where containment might just have a fighting chance. So that really corresponds to the earliest stages of the global spread, and, that's why we did all those things. And once we identify a suspected case, then of course, full infection control procedures in handling that particular passenger or visitor or patient in terms of transport to a designated hospital unit for quarantine plus or minus isolation.
>
> That was precisely forty days after May 1. And of course that's where the term quarantine comes from. So the border screening and all those containment-like measures at the earliest days, post–May 1, in my mind, allowed us to delay the community spread, or extensive community seeding. Precisely for the period that the ancients had in mind, forty days. So you quarantine and you buy ten days. And my colleagues at the university studied this and mathematically showed that this was true. Most of the literature will tell you that border screening does not work, if your objective is to completely stop the introduction of infectious seeds. But what the literature also shows is that you can buy a few weeks, you can delay it a few weeks, and those few weeks could be quite crucial in terms of ramping up your community response in mitigation.
>
> And if you look at the sociology and the population psychology, as a result of the 1997 H5N1 outbreak here, and the 2003 SARS outbreak, I think not having those initial containment-like measures, including school closures, would have been untenable. But of course not every population or society has the infrastructure, has the logistics, capabilities, and the population readiness to implement and support these interventions. So I'm not here to say that, universally, that is what every society or population ought to have done. What I'm saying is that it's a highly contextual decision, and that in our context, it was the right thing to do. And I remain of that view.

Hong Kong's decision to quarantine is initially explained here in relationship to its past experience with SARS and its unique policy of continual temperature screening at its borders. Professor Leung also locates Hong Kong within a global framework by arguing that containment is in agreement with WHO recommendations for early stages of an influenza pandemic. The proffered rationale for extending quarantine for a full forty-day period is then connected both to "what the ancients had in mind"—part of an argument related to historical precedent—and to scientific data that suggests that containment measures allowed Hong Kong to "buy time," to delay the widespread infection by a measure of days or weeks—part of an argument related to hard science. Lastly, Professor Leung effectively argues that the "context" of Hong Kong—with its unique social and psychological characteristics—should not be ignored when making epidemiological decisions about the type of response that is "appropriate." Like Dr. Tsang, Professor Leung suggests that Hong Kong's citizens demand quarantine, that they expect it, and that it is effective for delaying the spread of disease.

In interviews with other experts working in Hong Kong, I was repeatedly assured that containment measures such as quarantine, border screening, and school closures were effective, despite what others outside the SAR might conjecture. Dr. Ben Cowling, an epidemiologist working at the University of Hong Kong, argued that his data show clearly that entry screening might delay the start of a local epidemic by one or two weeks. Musing on the use of quarantine for flu, Cowling said: "I think that other containment efforts, like aggressive contact tracing and quarantine, would also add a similar amount. I don't have any data on that, but that's my suspicion: it can buy you on the order of a week, maybe two weeks. But it can't buy months. You can't keep out flu, but you can delay it." A similar viewpoint was expressed by Malik Peiris, the co-discoverer of SARS, who suggested that "In retrospect, it probably delayed the takeoff of the peak of the outbreak in Hong Kong. There's no way of really knowing. But I think the mathematical modeling experts probably have some insight into it. But my gut feeling is that it probably did delay that May introduction." Off the record, another internationally recognized epidemiologist working in Hong Kong told me that containment measures like quarantine were possible only in a place like China—a nation that had the political power and the will to act quickly and aggressively to halt a pandemic. He argued that "In a severe pandemic, *there will be winners and losers*. It would have been terrible if, for a couple of weeks, you'd let it [the H1N1 virus] go in the US and then realized that it was more severe and there was no other option, because other countries were already controlling or mitigating."

While working inside the CDC during the fall of 2009, I attended a talk on China's public health capacity given by Wang Yu, the director of the Chinese CDC. As part of his talk, Wang Yu likewise explained that China's drastic border control measures during the 2009 H1N1 pandemic were a way to "buy time." He argued that China had few material supplies for a response (no stockpile of Tamiflu or other prophylactic drugs) and that therefore the Chinese authorities had felt it was necessary to instead slow the spread of the virus through a combination of border control, quarantine, and isolation of confirmed cases. Wang Yu argued, in effect, that since China had relatively little capacity compared to the West, its top priority would always be prevention. It was always better, he said, to "hope for the best, but prepare for the worst." The meaning was clear; Wang Yu was arguing his case for the Chinese policy of containment in addition to mitigation for influenza.

Elsewhere, Dr. Thomas Tsang has openly argued that Hong Kong is "an epidemiological window to what happens in mainland China." He also positions Hong Kong as a unique Chinese city, not just because of the fact that it borders mainland China, but also as a "result of its separate, independent health administration." Both of these points were apparent throughout my various conversations about H1N1 in Hong Kong and mainland China. However, Dr. Tsang has also written that he believes mainland China is Hong Kong's "most important strategic partner" in the control of infectious disease. (Tsang 2009, 83, 85.) I want to stress here that Dr. Tsang's willingness to give primacy to Hong Kong's relationship with China over that with the international community is crucial to understanding Hong Kong's developing role in emergent global networks. It signals that, at least on an epidemiological level, Hong Kong thinks of itself as being closer to China than to its other national partner agencies (such as the CDC). And, perhaps indicative of this growing relationship, Hong Kong's official policy to quarantine was in agreement with the mainland's own decision to take extreme preventative measures during the 2009 pandemic. In an article on SARS, Leung has suggested that "internal politics" are often an issue during an epidemic, and remain an "outstanding problem for the Government" (2004, 75). In the case of the 2009 H1N1 pandemic, those politics were partially a result of Hong Kong's proximity to and growing relationship with the mainland. What interests me here is how experts in Hong Kong are able to negotiate between different "cultures" of public health in order to maintain local authority and undergird their global expertise.

In Hong Kong, universal ideas about the effectiveness of containment are tested empirically, socially, and politically. Hong Kong's experts use the idea of local context to their best advantage and to undergird their own expertise. The meaning and uses of quarantine in Hong Kong are, in fact, always negotiable. Hong Kong's decision to quarantine during the first wave of the H1N1 pandemic was grounded in solid epidemiological reasoning—in a scientific logos that could be universally agreed upon. In interviews, epidemiologists repeatedly pointed out to me that Hong Kong's judgments were based on a local analysis of international events and upon the information that was circulating during April, May, and June of 2009. For my part, I want to stress the use of the "local picture" in the views quoted above as it relates to the translation of international information as circulated by the WHO. Hong Kong officials, much like their counterparts in the United States or the UK, must take local context into account in order to make any sense out of globally circulating information. However, because Hong Kong is already conceived of as self-contained and "unique" (located both physically and ideologically in between the Chinese and Western systems), it has a greater flexibility to choose a course of action that fits with its local history, circumstances, and events.

"It's Mostly Political": Quarantine from a Western Perspective

Outside of Hong Kong and China, the standard viewpoint on using containment measures for influenza is that they don't work. Quarantine is still seen as an effective public health response measure for outbreaks of infectious diseases, but what works against microbes such as SARS, MERS (Middle East Respiratory Syndrome), or Ebola will not work for the influenza virus.[13] Hong Kong's decision to quarantine was often interpreted as being a political decision, based on an emotional reaction to its past experiences with SARS, or as a particularly Chinese decision.

An epidemiologist working in a regional WHO office explained Hong Kong's response as being in step with China's. Both, she said, had taken "very aggressive stances to H1." She explained that the decisions to quarantine, border-screen, and close schools were based partly on political grounds and partly on their experiences with H5N1 and SARS. She argued that the Chinese think "of containment as a very severe slowdown, and they've just published a paper on how effective these measures have been." She went on to suggest that "They've clearly got some 'end goal' in mind, but we've not discussed it with them as such. They really don't want to make the same mistakes that they made with SARS. Their political pain with SARS was enormously felt in China, so they're willing to take a risk on overly aggressive measures for containment." For many, Hong Kong's actions were seen, as one UK epidemiologist best expressed it, as "somewhere in between China and the rest of the world." These viewpoints are expressive of Hong Kong's positioning as being between China and the West. To borrow from scholar Richard Madsen, Hong Kong—like China—is always enmeshed in "debates about central common meanings." In terms of its response, then, Hong Kong is seen here as not following "the plot of the master story" being told about the 2009 pandemic by those outside of China. (Madsen 1995, 211, 162.) At stake is the common meaning of the epidemiological effectiveness of quarantine, which is thus situated in the context of its use as well as its scientific rationale.

A top virologist working in the United States described Hong Kong's and China's decision to quarantine in a similar vein. To him, mainland China's decision was based on its population size and its minimal resources, not necessarily on sound epidemiological data on quarantine's effectiveness. He explained that "They really don't have many options. They are not going to have antivirals available and they don't have much flu vaccine capacity. A lot of it is political, but they also see that they don't have many options." Hong Kong, on the other hand, was described as having a "tremendous public health system, good disease and animal surveillance— almost better than any other country." Hong Kong's decision to quarantine, unlike China's, was related to its experience with SARS and its small, densely concentrated population, which meant that containment *might* work in Hong Kong to delay the spread of the virus. Another epidemiologist concurred with this viewpoint and told me that Hong Kong's experts had pressed their US counterparts to be more aggressive in their response. Many experts in Hong Kong had indeed expressed to me a low-level frustration that the United States had not done more to contain the spread of the virus during the early weeks of its own outbreak. This was also seen by

Hong Kongers as being political in nature—suggesting to me that quarantine would not work in the United States because it was neither politically feasible nor socially palatable.

While working at the CDC, I often heard various epidemiologists and virologists express a longing to obtain China's level of authority in times of emergency. Scientists trained in the Western tradition often internalize the so-called norms of science: communalism, univeralism, disinterestedness, originality, and skepticism. Within this Mertonian framework, the practice of science is conceptually linked to the practice of democracy—at least in theory (see Brown 2009 for an examination of the historical relationship between science, expertise, and democracy). Most US and European experts expressed a conviction that decision-making during a pandemic should be made scientifically and democratically. And yet these underlying cultural assumptions were often openly questioned whenever the topic of quarantine was raised. Temporary authoritarianism, many Western epidemiologists mused in private, would be a boon during any crisis situation when decisions needed to be made quickly in order to protect the general population.

Many experts I interviewed who worked in global health conceptualized Hong Kong as having the best of both worlds during any pandemic: access to Western methods of disease prevention and outbreak response and Chinese political authority to act without waiting for democratic approval. As one US expert put it: "I *wish* we could quarantine here without interference. Or force people to get vaccinated. That would be terrific in terms of stopping a deadly pandemic." Another epidemiologist working in the United States lamented that Hong Kong and China were "capable of doing things that other countries aren't able to do" from either a financial or a political standpoint. Quarantine costs a lot of money. It requires people's cooperation. Containment measures not only interrupt the flow of viruses, they stop the flow of goods and people and have the potential to throw financial markets into disarray. From the perspective of those working outside of Asia, China quarantined not only because it believed containment measures delayed the start of an outbreak, but because it could.

Hong Kong as Weather Vane

Debates over the effectiveness of quarantine, its political and epidemiological uses, and its conceptualization as a particularly "Chinese" response to outbreaks of infectious disease, are all indicative of the impact of geography, history, and "culture"—a combination that tended to be glossed as *local context* by the epidemiologists I interviewed or worked with—on the practice of global public health. "Universal" best practices during a pandemic are thus highly negotiable; the meanings of quarantine are always variable. The interpretation of epidemiological science depended, at least in part, on the past experiences and local circumstances of the experts involved. Hong Kong's postcolonial temporality—its history and geographical position—matters to the construction and enactment of viral expertise in the territory.

What's more, Hong Kong's containment measures were seen by outside experts as somehow revealing its growing identification as a Chinese city. The significant role that Hong Kong continues to play within global influenza and infectious disease surveillance, research, and response networks—as a key node in the superorganism of global public health—means that Hong Kong's actions matter to the development and creation of universal scientific knowledge about influenza and epidemiological responses to burgeoning global outbreaks of novel strains of the flu. History and geography and "culture" matter to the creation of epidemiological knowledge and viral expertise.

In the next chapter, we will see how the 1997 H5N1 outbreak in Hong Kong epitomizes the very idea of a global flu pandemic. Recent "bird flu" narratives connecting the H5N1 virus to the deadly 1918 pandemic of H1N1 loop between past and future not only in order to undergird the need for continued scientific research funding for Influenza A surveillance but to garner international support for global pandemic preparedness in general. Thus we will see how an outbreak in Hong Kong came to represent all future outbreaks; the Sirens' song of influenza knowledge and preparedness has its origins in postcolonial temporality.

4

THE SIREN'S SONG OF AVIAN INFLUENZA

A Brief History of Future Pandemics

I think there are two camps: "we're all going to die," and "there's nothing to
worry about and we don't want to overreact," or "I've got my bird flu plan."
But that didn't help with this outbreak. We were too H5 focused, so that
when we got this shift, we were uncertain about where to go.

An epidemiologist working in a local Department
of Public Health in California

Gene Segment HA. Biological function: *The hemagglutinin gene segment encodes for a surface protein on the influenza virus responsible for attaching it to
the host cell. It recognizes the appropriate receptor proteins on the surface of cells
and then effectively binds the virus to the host. Changes in the genetic makeup
of this segment are closely monitored through surveillance, as any alteration
has the potential to affect Influenza A's infectivity and virulence.* Pathographic
function: *This chapter analyzes the various historical, biological, and social
narratives that bind the 1997 H5N1 outbreak to the 1918 H1N1 pandemic to
the 2009 H1N1 pandemic. The result of this merging of time/space—in which
the H5N1 virus is transformed into the representative infectious disease agent
at the heart of most pandemic planning—is the concept of "bird flu" itself. In
effect, this chapter examines how history and biology combine to produce an
infective trope of a deadly future influenza pandemic; a specter that is then used
effectively by experts to ground further global research, surveillance, and planning programs.*

As late as the summer of 2012, experts involved in the 2009 H1N1 response—social scientists, virologists, epidemiologists, and public health officials alike—continued to share and gather tales of the pandemic. Throughout workshops and debriefings that I observed or guided in my role as a consultant, people rehashed events and decisions in order to comprehend something beyond any individual ken. Maybe if we pooled our resources, the collective logic seemed to go, we might be able to grasp at a larger truth about the effectiveness of and gaps in global public health systems and preparedness. In trying to reconstruct the global pandemic, in all the retellings of its smaller local or national events, we found ourselves grappling with notions of uncertainty and risk (for more on the role uncertainty played in 2009, see chapter 5), problems related to open access to "actionable" information (for more on the problem of the "data deluge," see chapter 6), and the constant, overhanging threat that we might all be eventually either lulled into a false sense of security or pushed into a heightened state of anxiety by listening to *too many* narratives about influenza. In this chapter, I will argue that viruses like influenza hold the promise of ultimate biological knowledge reminiscent of the Greek myth of the Sirens' song, and just as distracting.

Ironically, the Sirens are first depicted as half-human and half-bird—portrayed in early Greek art with the head of a woman and a bird's body and legs. Divine beings who lived on an island in the sea, their singing was so delicious to the ears of men that any who sailed past their island were certain to be lured to their deaths. At their clawed feet lay heaps of skeletal remains, human remnants of those who had heeded the Sirens' call and never returned. The Sirens make two main appearances in Greek mythology: once when Orpheus saves Jason and the Argonauts from sure destruction by playing his lyre to drown out their voices, allowing the Argonauts to safely sail past the island; and again in the *Odyssey*, when the cunning goddess Circe helps Ulysses to escape the Sirens' call by enjoining him to pack his crew's ears with wax. Circe tells Ulysses that he can listen to the song himself so long as he instructs his men to tie him firmly to the mast of their ship and to ignore all his pleas to be unfastened. As they sail past, Ulysses hears the Sirens singing. Edith Hamilton, in her seminal work, *Mythology*, tells us that it was the words of their song that were the most enticing and maddening. The Sirens' song promised knowledge far beyond man's ken, "ripe wisdom and a quickening of the spirit" (Hamilton 1963, 214). Hamilton asserts that it was this promise of godlike knowledge that lured men to their deaths, not the sheer beauty of the song itself. With access to the Sirens' information, anyone would be able not only to see into the future but to know all things. In other words, all who heard the song would be consummately prepared to act to their best advantage. No wonder, then, that two thousand years after first heard their invitation, the concept of the Sirens' song remains so compelling.

In *The Dialectic of Enlightenment*, Max Horkheimer and Theodor Adorno use the Sirens' song as an allegory for man's desire to triumph over brute nature using scientific reason. For Horkheimer and Adorno, the Sirens' song is representative of an alluring past that threatens to return Ulysses back to a primitive state (2002, 26). The tale of Ulysses and the Sirens, then, is ultimately about the triumph of the mind over art, reason over nature, objectivity over subjectivity, the future over the past. But if Hamilton's view is accurate, the Sirens' song does not just contain all past knowledge, as Horkheimer and Adorno suggest, but all future knowledge as well. The song, then, is enticing because it is *pure knowledge*. It promises a knowledge that allows a perfect rationality; to hear the song is to be able to choose the perfect course of *action*. That is why the myth of the Sirens' song is so perfectly suited to unpacking the various narratives—expert, scientific, personal, cultural, and political—surrounding influenza. Influenza captures the attention of scientists, epidemiologists, public health policy planners, politicians, journalists, and ordinary citizens alike. Its call beckons us into an uncertain future but promises that the knowledge it contains might save us. And yet, as much as the Sirens promise Ulysses "to sing of 'everything,'" in reexamining Homer's original narrative one notices that the Sirens ultimately "sing of nothing other than the fact that they are to sing: a song about itself" (Comay 2000, 36). The Sirens' song, then, is about all future songs; it is the promise of knowledge without the knowledge itself, the choice not necessarily to act but to gather better information to inform future actions.

The promise of ultimate knowledge that the mythological song contains is a ripe allegory for analyzing the modern-day search for scientific knowledge and the promises which such knowledge seems to contain. The various scientific narratives spun about influenza ultimately reflect the larger epidemiological quest for actionable knowledge *before* any infectious disease pandemic gets under way, flu or not. If we could stop or predict a deadly novel influenza strain before it truly begins, then we might understand enough about all viruses to stop other deadly infectious disease outbreaks. In fact, many experts argue that this is the only way to prevent another deadly pandemic such as the infamous one caused by an H1N1 Influenza A virus in 1918, estimated to have killed up to forty million people,[1] and whose specter continues to haunt (and to taunt) public health. The influenza virus, then, holds out an almost mythlike promise to epidemiologists and virologists everywhere. This chapter, then, is an attempt to unravel the song from its promise, to examine the ways in which the lure of scientific knowledge about deadly strains of influenza steered the ship of public health slightly off course.

The metaphor of the Sirens' song echoes in my analysis below of the different, but overlapping, narratives about influenza, in particular "bird flu." Until the outbreak of H7N9 in 2013, H5N1 was the subtype of Influenza A most commonly referenced as "bird flu" by both the media and experts. The generally accepted stories about the origins of H5N1 from a scientific perspective mirror the more recent cultural, institutional, and political narratives concerning pandemic influenza (or "pan flu") and preparedness told from a macroscopic perspective. Narratives about pan flu are always threefold: biological, historical, and social. Retold in juxtaposition or in close relationship to each other, these layered narratives about H5N1 craft a modern mythical tale about a deadly scourge that never was but soon will be. Stories about pan flu form the basis for a greater understanding of the political ramifications of the global 2009–10 H1N1 pandemic response (as will be discussed in more detail throughout the following two chapters).

In 2009, these narratives mattered more than ever; they aided both experts and "laypeople" in attempts to understand events that never seemed to have a clear-cut beginning or ending. At different locations and times throughout the pandemic, stories I heard and read about influenza seemed to all lack a certain "narrative coherence" (Liu 2002, 102). It was not that the epidemiologists and scientists I talked with did not recollect what actually occurred during the early days and weeks of 2009 or could not tell me "the story," but rather that they often had difficulty narrating smaller instances or moments of decision-making in any kind of "meaningful temporal sequence" (Liu 2002, 102). Their oral retellings of events often jumped back and forth in time and space, with moments and information all linked together like some kind of aural hypertext (or, to loop back to the last chapter, a type of postcolonial temporality). To understand what was happening as it unfolded in 2009, public health experts often shared stories of their experience with past outbreaks of influenza or SARS in an effort to place uncertain epidemiological information back into some context or relationship to known facts. The stories that people told me were often filled with details that were meant to recreate for me the anxiety, excitement, and frenetic energy of the first few weeks of the pandemic. They were also, as I would come to understand much later, representative of each individual's attempts to better understand and analyze events and actions. Even in 2013, as this book was being revised, stories about the 2009 H1N1 pandemic were, at least from the perspective of a traditional narrative arc, still unfinished.

The unfinished epidemiological narratives about H5N1, H7N9, and H1N1 explored in this chapter are ultimately a type of "technology" (Wald 2008, 19) that crafts and binds together entire populations through the trope of susceptibility. Seen through this lens, tales of a future H5N1 pandemic have helped to construct a truly "global" public health, one in which we see "communicability configuring community" (Wald 2008, 12) on a global scale. Throughout the 2009 H1N1 pandemic, discussions about bird flu's relationship to the circulating virus (both in print and in speech) were at least partially constitutive of the events themselves.[2] Ultimately, I argue that over a decade of prior research, focus on the Influenza A subtype known as H5N1 was as important to the collective understanding of the 2009 pandemic as the H1N1 virus itself.

PANDEMIC!!! The Continually Reemergent Story

Tracking the beginnings—or origins—of our modern fascination with and fear of influenza is, at best, difficult to do. Influenza is an old disease. So, too, our fears about it. Looking specifically at how bird flu came to be at the center of our imaginings about the future shape and scale of pandemics requires that we have flexible concepts of time and space. This is not a linear story that I'm about to tell; past and future collide together in the space of the present. The 1918 swine flu and the future possibility of a bird flu pandemic both played an equal part in how the 2009 H1N1 virus was conceptualized. In order to track back and forth from 1918 to the future to 2009 and back again, I borrow philosopher Mikhail Bakhtin's concept of the "chronotope" or "time space." In the chronotope, time is "thickened" and space is "responsive to the movements of time" (Bakhtin 1981, 84). To examine how the specter of a global bird flu pandemic influenced preparedness planning in public health and inflected the 2009 H1N1 response, I turn first to an analysis of how our conception of bird flu was shaped by the influenza pandemic of 1918.

Ultimately, and following historian William Cronon, I suggest here that "to recover the narratives people tell themselves . . . is to learn a great deal about their past actions and about the way they understand those actions. Stripped of the story, we lose track of understanding itself" (Cronon 1992, 1369). Without examining the various narratives that people continuously tell about the influenzas of 1918 and 1997, we risk losing a critical part of our understanding of the actions public health experts took during the 2009 H1N1 outbreak. The ultimate effect of the rhetorical entanglement of past influenzas with present-day strains was to erase differences between very distinct influenza viruses, different eras, and discrete places. In essence, public health experts used familiar narratives about 1918 and 1997 to help them make decisions in 2009.

In what follows, I explore how the 1918 H1N1 became linked to the 1997 H5N1 which then became the basis not only for pandemic influenza plans but for fears about the circulating H1N1 subtype in 2009. This past-present-past-future-past looping created a chronotope wherein an influenza pandemic is ever-emergent and ever-present. The 1918 H1N1 Influenza A strain was often discursively entwined with the 1997 H5N1 and the 2009 H1N1 influenza A strains in three overlapping, yet distinct, narratives: biological, historical, and what I will label as "prophetic past-future." And yet, as epidemiologist Stephen S. Morse writes in the preface to the 1993 volume *Emerging Viruses*: "Despite our wish to anticipate emerging diseases, we cannot foretell the future. What we can do is to draw the best inferences possible from past experience; for this, history can be a valuable guide" (viii).

It is the history of the 1918 pandemic that I turn to next, paying particular attention to how the 1918 virus has been used to construct a future H5N1 pandemic. The history of the 1918 virus not only bleeds into our conceptualization of avian influenza but also contaminates our thinking about possible future pandemics. Since 1997, the historical narrative of 1918 has transformed into the unfinished story of H5N1.

The History/Narrative of 1918

In March 1918, when influenza first broke out among US Army troops stationed in Kansas, World War I had already been raging for three and a half long years. The outbreak of flu, while noted, went largely unremarked until the so-called second wave of the pandemic hit the United States in the fall of that same year. Influenza seems to have been brought back to the country via returning troops aboard a naval vessel that docked in New York City. A newspaper story from October 6, 1918, chronicles one day in the fight against influenza. The *New York Times*'s headline reports sixty-one deaths the day before—an increase over the day before that—and details a new work hours timetable with a listing of shop and school closures. The city requisitioned hospitals in preparation for a large increase in influenza cases and yet the overall tone of the article is confident, not panicked or overly anxious. A spokesperson for the city Health Department is quoted as stating: "I believe the epidemic can be handled without its alarming spread" (*New York Times* 1918). Yet spread it did. In the United States, the "Spanish flu" caused widespread illness and an alarming rate of death in young people (defined as between the ages of twenty and forty). By the end of the third wave of the pandemic, an estimated forty million people worldwide would be dead from influenza and its complications (Taubenberger and Morens 2006, 15).

Scholars who study the 1918 influenza are often puzzled by the relative lack of attention paid to the pandemic—both at the time and for decades afterward. Historian Alfred Crosby refers to it as the "forgotten pandemic" in the title of his recent book on the subject (2003). And yet, as journalism professor Debra Blakely has shown in her recent analysis of over eight hundred *New York Times* articles written about and during the 1918, 1957, and 1968 influenza pandemics, the 1918 pandemic was not—as has been suggested elsewhere—"forgotten" or "ignored" (2003). The newspaper's coverage of the pandemic, according to Blakely, "changed daily," relied heavily on war metaphors to describe public health measures being taken to stave off spread, and depicted officials as "not in control" of the situation. Stories put the blame for influenza equally on health and government officials. Once deaths from influenza disappeared, so did the news stories. Interestingly, the 1918 pandemic was only labeled as such post hoc—long after deaths had subsided. Before that, throughout the outbreaks and despite reports of influenza worldwide, events during 1918 were referred to as an epidemic. During subsequent pandemics, newspaper articles directly referred to that of 1918 as "the cause for alarm and risk." (Blakely 2003, 889, 893.) So if, as it appears from Blakely's analysis, the 1918 pandemic was reported upon and was never forgotten, what are we to make of its resurgence in the 1970s as a subject for serious academic research and in the 2000s as a topic able to garner both public and expert attention?

Public health scholar Philip Alcabes, in his book *Dread*, discusses how the "Spanish flu" of 1918 was all but forgotten by researchers and nonfiction writers alike (though not by novelists such as Katherine Anne Porter) until the 1970s, when it was resurrected by epidemiologists and virus specialists "who were interested in promoting their theory that devastating flu outbreaks occur every decade or so." Going further, Alcabes argues: "Today, all discussions of flu involve some retrospection on the Spanish Flu epidemic, the rationale for 'pandemic preparedness.' There is an imagined epidemic that carries meanings not self-evident in the original event" (Alcabes 2009, 6). To put it another way, the story of 1918 has been decontextualized from its original meaning and recontextualized (Bauman and Briggs 1990) within present narratives about H5N1 (or, more recently, H7N9) to create an imagined pandemic. It is to this partially reimagined history and wholly imagined future, then, that I turn to next and which will undergird much of the rationale and rethinking for public health response to the 2009 H1N1 pandemic.

The Legacy of 1918

As historian of public health Charles Rosenberg once argued, we are prepared to fear what we have been prepared to see (Rosenberg and Golden 1992, 186). The history of the 1918 pandemic prepared scientists to see—and to fear—the H5N1 outbreak in 1997. It is impossible to say how public health experts might have assessed the threat in the absence of 1918. That is an unworkable conjecture; 1918 has totally saturated the ways in which we conceive of pandemic influenza. So much so that influenza experts conceive of the 1918 virus as the "mother of all pandemics" (Taubenberger and Morens 2006).

Washington Post journalist Alan Sipress links 1918 to H5N1 in the preface to his book on avian influenza, ultimately arguing that "today we remain closer than we've ever been to a repeat of the Great Influenza of 1918." Sipress reconstructs a conversation he had with Keiji Fukuda, the WHO's Director of Influenza, who explains his own experience during the early outbreaks of H5N1, telling Sipress that "it really brought us back to 1918." (Sipress 2009, 6, 68.) The language used by Fukuda here is especially interesting in that it transports us in time and space. The past here is compressed into the present and stretched out into the future. Indeed, 1918 is often discursively linked to the threat of a future avian influenza pandemic through the specter of H5N1.

However, the 1918 influenza pandemic has not always been of immediate concern to either the public or public health officials (the exception, as highlighted in the section above, being the successive influenza pandemics in 1957 and 1968). The 1918 pandemic was, as it were, rediscovered as a focal point for both anxiety and intensive scientific research. It reemerged along with our fears about calamitous future influenza outbreaks. Pete Davies discusses the lack of funding for influenza prior to 2000 and how experts at the CDC lament that influenza isn't as exciting or fund-worthy as something like HIV (2000). Davies's book is about the search for the 1918 virus in frozen bodies buried deep in the tundra near the Arctic Circle. The 1918 virus is the ultimate Siren in this narrative; it is hoped that by understanding the H1N1 strain that killed millions, scientists might learn something about H5N1. In a book on H5N1, Mike Davis reports that interest in 1918 amped up in 1974, only a few years before the 1976 swine flu pandemic. Davis suggests that pre-1918, flu was "not considered a serious killer" and argues that the memory of 1918 was "repressed" because it was a failure of science. (Davis 2005, 24, 32, 33.) But was the memory of 1918 repressed or was the event itself just forgotten until it was revived by epidemiologists working on influenza in the latter half of the twentieth century?

In her influential book, *The Coming Plague*, journalist Laurie Garrett highlights how the historical influenza pandemic of 1918 influenced decision-making during the 1976 swine flu outbreak. As she argues, public health officials believed that the consequences of being wrong about the severity of the 1976 virus would be devastating. Although pandemic predictions, as one top epidemiologist explained it, were like "weather forecasts" and "hazardous business," public health experts ultimately decided to err on the side of caution (Garrett 1994, 159–60). The resultant vaccines produced in 1976 caused several cases of Guillain–Barré Syndrome[3] and cost millions of dollars. Ultimately, the scandal caused by the so-called overreaction to the 1976 swine flu would continue to be balanced by fears about a repeat performance of 1918. By 2009, public health officials had become trapped in a need to triangulate between 1918, 1976, and 2003 (the year of the SARS outbreak); it would not be easy to see 2009's influenza outbreak clearly or objectively.

In his book about the 1918 virus, Davies begins the story of the infamous pandemic with a chapter on the 1997 H5N1 outbreak in Hong Kong. In it, the influenza virus is described as a "terrorist." Robert Webster is quoted as being convinced that the H5N1 viral outbreak in Hong Kong in 1997 was like the 1918 H1N1. Keiji Fukuda was also concerned that the situation with H5N1 was similar—too similar—to H1N1. (Davies 2000, 9, 35, 36.) The linking of the two viruses is not accidental, nor is it necessarily evidentiary. The viruses were two different subtypes of the same class of Influenza A viruses, but they were not the same virus. And yet, putting them in juxtaposition caused H5N1 to take on the rhetorical casting of the "new" 1918 H1N1. This was the "same" or a similar threat in a new guise. This type of thinking makes a stronger response to the threat of H5N1 (or any other novel influenza) all the more likely.

The Institute of Medicine utilizes influenza as a case study in how the US system is unprepared for large outbreaks or pandemics. In a pull-out box in *Microbial Threats to Health: Emergence, Detection, and Response*, the specific case of the 1918 influenza pandemic is used to highlight the threat of future pandemics and the need to remake the virus using reverse genetics technology in order to learn more about viral pathogenicity. The institute stresses that a future pandemic is "inevitable" and "overdue," but that—despite pandemic planning—we "remain poorly prepared." (1992, 136–38.) Scholar Gerald Callahan's book on infections (2006) also links the story of 1918 to the threat of a future H5N1 pandemic in a chapter named after influenza's nickname, "The Slate Wiper." The name refers to influenza's ability to "wipe out" millions of humans in one wave, thus "cleaning the slate."

Books targeted at a general audience also seem to tap into this modern fear of bird flu as a "disaster" waiting to happen. In the early 2000s, one medical doctor was so concerned with news reports of avian influenza that he decided to self-publish three separate books on the topic. He argues that we are "in denial" about the threat of bird flu and suggests his books are an attempt to spur action. Woodson avowedly wants to frighten people into preparing for what is, in his opinion, a certain catastrophe (Woodson and Jodrey 2005, 4, 10). The books also rhetorically and scientifically connect the 1918 H1N1 virus to the H5N1 virus, pushing readers to see H5N1 as akin to the worst known pandemic influenza in history. Other authors writing for a general audience take great pains not only to map out what "will" happen during a pandemic, but how to prepare for societal collapse and panic (Fonte 2006, Greene 2006). A slightly more tongue-in-cheek book entitled *The Little Book of Pandemics: 50 of the World's Most Virulent Plagues and Infectious Diseases* (Moore 2007), lists influenza and H5N1 bird flu as plagues number one and two, respectively.

Published in the wake of outbreaks of H5N1 in 2005, such fear-mongering books all capitalize on our collective anxiety about another 1918-sized pandemic by purporting to prepare or educate us for the next "big one." While some are more scientific and scholarly than others, all of these popular accounts of influenza resonate with apprehension on the part of actual scientists and officials about future influenza outbreaks. Things might work out, but then again, they might not. H5N1 could just disappear or become a nonissue; or bird flu could become more deadly and capable of person-to-person transmission and kill up to 30 percent of the global population. Caught between the poles of 1918 and 1997, these authors all suggest that their readers must collectively decide what the real threat or risk posed by H5N1 is. The H5N1 virus is a symbol here of the potential for influenza to decimate the human population. It prepares us to fear, as Rosenberg suggests, what we have been prepared to see.

By the end of journalist Sipress's book on avian influenza, the more recent 2009 H1N1 pandemic has officially begun. After years of chasing after the Siren song of bird flu, it should come as no surprise when officials like the WHO's general director Margaret Chan make specific recourse to the H5N1 threat in their calls to action in 2009 (Sipress 2009, 327). As Sipress's account highlights—and the last section of this chapter will show—the echo of two decade's worth of fears about H5N1 reverberated throughout the early days of the 2009 H1N1 response. The next section examines how the 1918 and avian influenza strains are interwoven with the 2009 H1N1 virus not only in historical terms, but in biological ones. Biological narratives here link the viral past to the viral future through a viral present.

Connecting Viruses in 1918, 1997, and 2009

Biologically speaking, all pandemic influenza strains are somewhat related to each other, simply in the sense that all pandemic strains "ultimately acquired some or all of their gene segments from the avian IAV gene pool" (Morens and Taubenberger 2010, 327). Chapter 1 examined scientific attempts to understand something more about the class of Influenza A viruses through the construction of genetic phylogeny trees. By comparing the genetic sequences of influenza viruses, virologists hope to unravel the secrets of how viruses work, what makes them more or less pathogenic, transmissible, and deadly to humans. As the evolutionary virologists in chapter 1 caution, while genetic information can tell you a lot about where a virus came from, it cannot tell you much about where it is headed. But that fact doesn't necessarily stop public health experts from trying to extrapolate meaning from such genetic information. In the case of the 2009 H1N1 pandemic, experts wanted to know if the circulating virus shared similar genetic components to other, more deadly, influenza strains. Such knowledge was seen as providing partial answers to questions about how the 2009 H1N1 pandemic might develop, giving decisionmakers access to more actionable information.

Because little was known about the 2009 H1N1 virus, researchers immediately began "looking to the past for clues about the seasonality and geography of pandemic flu, the relationship between the new viruses and existing ones, and the behavior of this new H1N1's parent viruses in swine" (Cohen and Enserink 2009b, 996). A *Science* article published in early May 2009 reported that the 2009 H1N1 strain was "highly similar to a recently reconstructed human 1918 A (H1N1) virus and likely share[s] a common ancestor" (Garten et al. 2009, 197). Another article published in the same journal in May showed that the 2009 virus, despite a lingering and "substantial uncertainty," appeared to have less clinical severity than "the 1918 influenza pandemic but comparable with that seen in the 1957 pandemic." The authors duly warn in their conclusion that the "future evolution of the transmissibility, antigenicity, virulence, and antiviral resistance profile of this or any influenza virus is difficult to predict." (Fraser et al. 2009, 1557, 1561.) As CDC influenza expert Nancy Cox explained, these findings indicated that the 2009 virus ultimately did not seem to have the "markers of virulence that made the 1918 pandemic strain so deadly." Nevertheless, Cox went on to caution that there was "a great deal that we do not understand about the virulence of the 1918 virus or other viruses" (Silberner and Greenfieldboyce 2009).

One of the commonly discussed biological characteristics of influenza viruses is their ability to replicate much faster than other organisms. The evolutionary pace of H1N1 and H5N1—and, indeed, all Influenza A viruses—is impressively fast. The RNA of influenza is sometimes described as a "careless hack" whose copying mistakes lead to many errors in its millions of replications. These errors and the virus's high replication rate are the very reasons why flu evolves so rapidly. Because of this, influenza is often referred to as a "constantly emerging disease." (Davis 2005, 15, 11.) Influenza's rapid evolution is of concern to public health experts not only because a virus may quickly become more severe or deadly, but because of influenza's attendant facility in hiding from the human immune system, with its ability to develop antiviral resistance. Researchers sequence influenza viruses, in part, to better understand how viruses evolve into deadlier strains. After the 1918 pandemic strain was recovered from the lung tissue of a victim buried in tundra, it was sequenced for one main purpose: to discover what made it particularly catastrophic. Its genetic sequence was—and continues to be—compared to other, present-day virus strains. Sipress reports that influenza experts fear that, since its initial outbreak in 1997, "bird flu has become more like the Spanish flu strain" as it has evolved (2009, 69). The 1918 H1N1 strain has since become the model or standard for deadly flu strains; avian influenza viruses and the 2009 H1N1 virus were compared to the 1918 strain.

And yet, as with the reconstructed 1918 virus, researchers are no closer to understanding the biology of deadly influenza viruses like H5N1. The comparisons are, in essence, unavoidable, despite the lack of biological evidence to link them. As 1918 H1N1 is the only known catastrophic flu strain, what other comparisons—other than to that strain—are even conceivable? Researchers constantly admit that they don't know enough, or don't know much, about what makes any particular Influenza A strain highly pathogenic or easily transmissible. And as any evolutionary virologist will tell you, genetic markers that are associated with those traits are not necessarily the cause of them (see chapter 1). Correlation is not causation, despite the fact that the genetic makeup of influenza viruses seems to hold out an elusive key to better understanding of how viruses work or how they act "in the wild." As Sipress suggests: "Since the last pandemic in 1968, the revolutionary field of microbiology has indeed succeeded in breaking the genetic code of the microbes that menace us. But laboratory science has still failed to unlock the secrets of how this mercurial agent evolves and mutates, how it strikes its human prey and when" (2009, 239).

Microbiologist Paul Ewald points out the differences between warranted and unwarranted fears about influenza in his 2000 book, *Plague Time*. Warranted fears are due to the fact that certain groups—such as the elderly and children—are more vulnerable to infection and complications. Unwarranted fears stem directly from any comparison to the 1918 pandemic virus. Ewald explains that the rationale for looking for strains with similar hemagglutinin (HA) and neuraminidase (NA)—the two protein molecules that are most visible to the human immune system—is that they provide an easy comparison for virologists. Using them helps to narrow down the search for potentially deadly new strains. But as Ewald argues, similar HA and NA markers between the 1976 H1N1 pandemic strain—a mild one that caused little increase in normal flu fatality rates—and the 1918 H1N1 pandemic strain did not equate to a similarity in severity. Evolutionary virology, he argues, is not the same as biochemical science. As he explains: "The H1N1 marker had been present on dangerous viruses, but there was no reason to think that it made the viruses dangerous—with its high mutation rate, the influenza virus can generate tremendous variation within a matter of weeks while still retaining the same H1N1 marker." Going even further, he argues that modern-day influenza researchers do not use the "evolutionary perspective" correctly and "confuse similarity of hemagglutinin and neuraminidase molecules among different virus strains with similarities in the virulence of these strains." (Ewald 2000, 23, 25.) Despite this, virologists and epidemiologists alike turn to genetic information about viruses to help them understand something more about influenza. The RNA of Influenza A viruses—in particular that of the 1918 virus and the various H5N1 viruses that have been sequenced or genetically modified[4] since 1997—hold a particular fascination for scientists.

These viruses have become the modern-day Sirens of influenza re-searchers. Experts such as Taubenberger and Morens, in addition to label-ing the 1918 virus as the "mother of all pandemics," seek to understand something about the entire class of Influenza A viruses through careful study of the genetic makeup of the 1918 H1N1 virus and the evolution of its descendants. But, as we saw with the evolutionary virologists and their hesitation to use genetic markers to predict the future, knowing some-thing about the past 1918 or current H5N1 or H7N9 viruses does not mean knowing something about their potential futures. But this fact has not pre-vented experts from wishing it were not so and redoubling research efforts. As Taubenberger and Morens lament, scientists were "not much closer to understanding pandemic emergence in 2006 than we were in understand-ing the risk of H1N1 'swine flu' emergence in 1976" (2006, 21). Despite not knowing which genetic factors influence virus severity (or cause high mor-tality), scientists have kept listening to the Siren song of 1918 and H5N1. In 2009, years of focusing on 1918 and worrying about bird flu would come to a head during the first few weeks of a new influenza outbreak.

The Siren Song of H5N1

During the summer and fall of 2009, I often talked to epidemiologists try-ing to make sense of what had happened during the early days of the In-fluenza A (H1N1) outbreak that March. Their narratives of events slid back and forth from the present day to their past experiences with other outbreaks, such as SARS in 2003 and H5N1 in the years leading up to the pandemic. As Wittgenstein once noted, if all knowledge is based in expe-rience, then obviously it is our past experience that shapes our certainty about what we know in the present (1969, 35e). Science studies scholar Stephen Hilgartner suggests that events such as the 2009 H1N1 pandemic are not "objective occurrences" at all but rather actions that are constructed through the social dramas of the protagonists directly involved in them (2000, 148). Public health experts involved in the 2009 H1N1 response re-lied upon past experience to make decisions about the type of threat that the novel influenza virus posed. Knowledge of the 1918 pandemic and un-certainty about the threat of avian influenza impacted the ways in which public health experts could think about the 2009 influenza outbreak. It is in this sense that the 1918 and 1997 strains of influenza resemble the Sirens; the echoing voices of 1918 and 1997 lured the ship of global public health off its all-hazard course and onto the rocky shores of a milder-than-expected Level 6 influenza pandemic.

An article in *Nature*, written in 2009 during the pandemic, suggested that public health systems were better prepared than they had been due to prior experience with SARS and pandemic planning for H5N1. But the article also admitted there had been "hiccups, due largely to the mismatch between pandemic scenarios envisaged and the one that has arrived." For one, the 2009 pandemic was much milder than the ones most countries had initially planned for, which made the plans less useful for directing action. For another, most non-Asian countries had in place flu plans that conceived of potential threats spreading out of Southeast Asia. When the 2009 pandemic seemed to be developing instead in the United States and Mexico, it had public health officials scrambling to retool their responses. As the *Nature* article suggested, "officials were initially confused about how to implement response plans." That being said, planning for SARS and H5N1 did have some positive effects on the 2009 pandemic: the H1N1 virus was sequenced in record time; information was shared more readily and quickly post-SARS; and vaccines were in production much faster (Hayden 2009 passim, 756 [quotes]).

Throughout the fall of 2009, when I worked inside the CDC, I continually asked people about the early weeks of the response to the pandemic. By their pauses and measured answers, I could tell that some experts felt the initial public health response was less than perfect. A woman who had worked in the Emergency Operations Center (EOC) explained that it was as if no one knew what to do, despite the fact that people inside the agency had been running exercises and drills on the basis of H5N1 for a solid year before H1N1 broke out.

"It was like they all forgot that there were guidelines, that they had practiced everything," she said. "Look, you've got a plan. You know what you're supposed to do."

Her colleague, who had also worked in the EOC during the initial outbreak of H1N1, agreed with her, nodding as she explained that things seemed less organized, less practiced, than at her former job in the military—where people quite literally "knew the drill." In the Air Force, responsibilities during an emergency were known in advance; no one had to guess what their role would be or think about what to do—they just did it. That hadn't been the case with public health agencies. I told them that they were not alone, that several people from different organizations and agencies had expressed similar feelings and perspectives at debriefings on the pandemic I had attended. At one event, an expert from the WHO admitted she felt like everyone had "reinvented the wheel" when H1N1 happened.

The woman nodded and said, "Yes, that's it. But why? Why reinvent the wheel when you've got a plan right there? You should know what to do."

In point of fact, most public health agencies at the national and state levels not only had pandemic plans already in place, but had also extensively practiced for a future pandemic by running exercises based upon a fictional global outbreak caused by an infectious disease agent resembling H5N1 (a scenario itself partially modeled by using data on the 1918 H1N1 pandemic). Epidemiologists often saw these past exercises as having had positive and negative effects on the events of 2009. On one hand, prior pan flu drills had strengthened relationships among agencies and the individuals working in them; practicing responses to a pandemic had built greater trust between "partner" agencies. On the other hand, exercises and plans that had focused on an H5N1-type pandemic had left many experts feeling underprepared for actual events during the earliest weeks of the 2009 H1N1 outbreak. A flu expert working at the CDC remarked that "We had been preparing for many years for an H5 event, and we had a severity index in place for that, based on cases per death ratio. . . . So what was going on in Mexico, we really didn't have the denominator to calculate severity." A European vaccine research expert explained that before 2009 everyone was "sure" that bird flu would be the next pandemic, and much of the energy on vaccine development had been directed at preparing for H5N1 in particular. A communications expert at the US Department of Health and Human Services, presenting at a conference on H1N1, told the audience that, like everyone else, HHS had planned for the H5N1 virus, coming out of Asia, and thus had been surprised by an outbreak of H1N1 in Mexico. He joked to his (mostly expert) audience that viruses clearly didn't read flu plans. Events in 2009 underscored the need to retool plans based upon the H5N1 model. An expert working in Hong Kong expressed a hope that the lessons of 2009 would be packed back into global pandemic planning in order to strengthen future responses. By 2010, Hong Kong had already begun to revise its own local plans, he told me, and "the WHO is now undergoing a similar process—they are revising their pandemic plans. Because the current system under the WHO was designed with something like H5N1 in mind, without a factor to account for severity. So I think a new system incorporating severity would be very useful."

When I asked experts if they thought that the lessons from the 2009 pandemic had been learned, most replied in the positive. One of my coworkers at the CDC, Rohit Chitale, explored how past experience could affect action in the present. One of his superiors had watched a good friend die in a hospital in Hong Kong during SARS. Rohit thought that this event had colored the way that this person subsequently performed his job, the way that he envisioned public health's obligations and responsibilities. As Rohit explained, "It's personal for him. You can tell that he responds emotionally. He's seen it up close. I mean, here in the office, we see the reports, and few things scare us—we've seen such a wide range of things. After you've seen what we've seen, you don't get easily disturbed because we put things into the larger context, not focusing on anecdotes or patient-level experience. That's part of why we reacted slowly to H1^5—it just didn't seem all that bad in comparison. But for some people, it was different. Our boss—some of the other directors—they all thought this was 'the big one'—the global pandemic spread of H5."

At a meeting on influenza inside the CDC later that week, a flu expert maintained that if H1 had been H5, "We all would have been screwed." Someone else then joked that no one cared about H5 anymore. Another person across the room retorted, "It's waiting to bite us in the butt, though, don't worry." Then the entire room erupted in a brief spurt of laughter before going back to their discussion of internationally reported H1N1 case counts.

This insider joke belied the fact that H5N1 was the ghost in the pandemic planning machine. When it came to influenza strains, H5 was the scariest virus of them all. So much so that the virus had indeed become the basis for most public health planning efforts in the years leading up to 2009. As a top influenza expert explained in an effort to justify continued pandemic planning: "So many countries have influenza pandemic plans. It's not a new concept. The global community has benefitted from preparedness activities, simulations. Although they were painful, they were beneficial in helping to prepare us for an event like H1."

If the "working assessment was that this was severe," one expert had explained to me, then H5N1 had been part of the underlying rationale for assuming that the novel Influenza A (H1N1) virus would be severe. It wasn't all about biology, as another expert suggested in a meeting on the 2009 H1N1 response in July of that same year. She remarked that

> We prepared for the worst, but it wasn't as bad as we thought. There were political and legal aspects, the review of the pandemic plan was going on. Technically, if we were going by the books as they were published, we would have been at Level 6 in the first week. We didn't have the definition of sustained transmission, etc., and we had to improvise and were unable to give explanations. Being stuck in those phases just signaled our lack of— I don't know. In this case, we tried to go by the book. It was a political decision, it was not severity.

As this quote suggests, and as virologist Michael Oldstone has argued elsewhere: "The history of virology would be incomplete without describing the politics and the superstitions evoked by viruses and the diseases they cause." Fear and anxiety are "woven into the fabric of the history of viral plagues" (Oldstone 1998, 7). In this case, we might argue that fear and politics and the myth of a deadly H5N1 virus capable of sustained human-to-human transmission were woven into the fabric of pandemic influenza planning and disease outbreak planning in toto.

Nearly all the public health experts I interviewed reported feeling hamstrung by the pan flu plans that were already in place. Even if they had a gut feeling that H1N1 was not going to be a severe flu, the response system was not flexible enough to allow for any easy gradation of risk. All the plans were the same; the choice of responses was inflexible and based upon a severe influenza. An epidemiologist working in Europe expressed her personal opinion that there seemed little scientific rationality behind the WHO's response to the 2009 pandemic. Another epidemiologist based in the United States worried that the prior focus on H5N1 had been too "myopic." A leading influenza expert bemoaned that "what's always disappointed me is that there's all this focus on avian influenza" to the exclusion of other animal-based surveillance (such as surveillance of influenza circulating in pigs). The scientific evidence base for decision-making during an influenza outbreak, almost everyone I knew agreed, was very thin.

Most of the plans had been based on the conception of a future outbreak similar to H5N1, but had used 1918 as a model.

At a conference on the 2009 pandemic response, an epidemiologist working at the international level complained, "Our plans were drafted on the basis of the 1918 pandemic. Do we think of this as evidence-based?"

Another expert, responding to the question, said, "I don't think we have evidence for 1918, and that's why we've been modeling."

"And we are comfortable that the data for those models are good?" the first epidemiologist asked.

After a pause, another expert replied, "I think we're comfortable, but do we have proof? No."

Defending the 2009 response, an influenza expert from Europe said, "The pathogenicity of that virus [1918] was quite scary. We cannot say we don't have some element of evidence. It was different, but it's still valuable."

Other epidemiologists felt that the history of—or what was known about—the pandemic of 1918 was not a "controlled situation" (it had no possibility of having scientific controls on evidence) but gave public health experts some "perspective" on what might happen and what responses might be effective during a similarly severe pandemic. As a result, the plans based on scenarios created by using the 1918 H1N1 and 1997 H5N1 viruses as models weren't wrong per se, but needed to "evolve" along with the pathogen itself. One international expert suggested that the word "plan" was too restrictive; "guide" might have been a better term. No one expected public health experts to follow a plan exactly, but rather to use them creatively as a guide for action.

In essence, pandemic plans were used not only to shape actions but to defend them both ad and post hoc. Narratives about the 1918 pandemic and experiences during the SARS and H5N1 outbreaks were used to guide actions taken during the initial days of the 2009 H1N1 outbreak. As Jürgen Habermas has suggested: "Whenever agents use language to coordinate their actions, they enter into certain commitments to justify their actions (or words) on the basis of good reasons." These commitments, for Habermas, are validity claims, which have a "practical function" to "guide action" of social agents. Agents, such as the epidemiologists discussed here, are committed in advance to providing reasons for their actions during an event such as the 2009 pandemic and thus, these "reasons provide the invisible lines along which sequences of interactions unfold." For Habermas, one cannot know the meaning of an action unless one knows something about the subjectivity of the agent. Meaning, for Habermas, is intersubjective and not objective, and "shared meanings depend on shared reasons." (Finlayson 2005, 26, 27, 38, 35.) The public health experts above used stories about past and future pandemics to make commitments or stake validity claims about H1N1 in 2009.

Using the myth of Ulysses and the Sirens to talk about rational choice theory, scholar Jon Elster argues that "Societies as well as individuals have found it useful to bind themselves." Binding is an example of people "precommitting themselves" to a certain course of action. By binding themselves, in this case through the use of H5N1 pandemic planning, global public health experts thereby committed themselves to a very specific course of action during the 2009 pandemic. In essence, such acts of "investment" are often irreversible and commit the individuals to a preordained course of action that may cost them in the future. (Elster 1979, 37, 42.)

When the pandemic alarm was sounded in March of 2009, there was only one course of action for most public health experts to follow. Bound by pandemic plans set out in advance by the WHO and agreed upon by all member nations, public health institutions everywhere responded to the mild H1N1 pandemic *as if* it were H5N1. Once the emergency switch had been thrown, it was difficult—if not impossible—to change course. Actions set in motion by pandemic flu plans were carried out long after public health experts realized that the threat from H1N1 was relatively small. But this doesn't necessarily mean that pandemic planning itself was irresponsible or ineffective. As Elster suggests: "The Ulysses strategy is a precaution against inconsistency, not against irrationality; in fact it achieves consistency at the cost of an even larger departure from rationality." The choice to bind oneself ultimately depends on the value being placed on consistency over rationality (1979, 76). Borrowing from Elster, then, I suggest that the price of consistency in response action may have been too high during the 2009 H1N1 pandemic.

To really understand the meaning of actions taken during the pandemic in 2009, however, they must be put in juxtaposition to the history of 1918 and to the imagined future of an H5N1 pandemic. Epidemiologists working on the 2009 response constructed meaning around the novel H1N1 virus based on their shared experience and understanding of influenza. That experience included not only recent events such as the 1997 H5N1 outbreak, but knowledge of past events like the 1918 pandemic. But what kind of experience or meaning can be created from such narratives? In many ways, neither the pandemic of 1918 nor the possibility of a future H5N1 pandemic is ever "finished," and the stories we tell about 1918 and H5N1 are always unfinished narratives. And as they continuously unravel, they consciously and unconsciously drive global public health planning. An epidemiologist in Hong Kong put it thus: "I think that as a public health practitioner, you are only as good as your next epidemic, not your last epidemic. And I think, and to paraphrase Pasteur himself, chance favors the prepared mind. Just because we were prepared this time, perhaps that's why the heavens looked favorably on us. In terms of the biology of the bug and the clinical manifestations, H1N1 was not as severe or fatal as 1918. *But* that does not mean that the next time we're going to be as lucky." Such unfinished narratives of past outbreaks, however, work to partially craft the contours of all future outbreaks.

The Real Effect of Imagined Outbreaks: A Sirens' Song of Certain Risk and Ever-Present Uncertainty

The 1918 H1N1 virus and the elusive and enigmatic H5N1 virus are Sirens that continually sing promises of knowledge—and the possibility for action—to those working within global public health response today. Narratives continuously retold and reconstructed about the real, historical 1918 pandemic and the imagined, future H5N1 pandemic played a very real part in creating the 2009 H1N1 pandemic. In many ways, one cannot know about 2009 without recourse to the 1918 pandemic and the avian influenza outbreaks of 1997, 2003, and 2005. And yet how can one know something about a pandemic as it unfolds or has yet to be and—at least in the case of H5N1—has never been? How do public health experts calculate risk and take actions in the midst of such uncertainty? And, perhaps more importantly, how do we even know what we mean when we use the terms "risk" and "uncertainty" in relationship to influenza?

Scholars of science Michel Callon, Pierre Lascoumes, and Yannick Barthe are careful to articulate the differences between the concepts of risk and uncertainty in their book on decision-making in an increasingly uncertain world. Unhappy with the ways in which the two terms have been continuously conflated in modern parlance, they suggest that the term risk "designates a well-identified danger associated with a perfectly describable event or series of events." Risks have both objective and subjective probabilities that can be applied to known events: "The notion of risk is closely associated with that of rational decision." In other words, risk can be quantified and qualified. It is knowable. Since risk plays such a pivotal role in "rational choice," it should be reserved for use in situations where actors must choose between several paths of action. In contrast, uncertainty describes an entirely unknowable situation: "We know that we do not know, but that is almost all that we know: there is no better definition of uncertainty." In uncertain situations, then, one must decide without making a "definitive decision." In accordance with the "precautionary principle," precaution in relationship to uncertainty leads to "an active, open, contingent, and revisable approach. It is exactly the opposite of a clear-cut definitive decision." Callon and his colleagues want to be clear, however, about the difference between precaution and prevention. One needs to develop precaution in relationship to uncertainty; prevention is for coping with known risk. In effect, one cannot use prevention to think about uncertain events; for what would be prevented? (Callon, Lascoumes, and Barthe 2001, 19, 20, 21, 191, 192, 195.)

What's worse, expert knowledge—such as epidemiological reports that were broadcast throughout the media during the early days of the 2009 pandemic—can often lack the clarity necessary for communication of risk or uncertainty. Ludwik Fleck, writing about the production of scientific knowledge at the beginning of the twentieth century, asserted that "Certainty, simplicity, vividness originate in popular knowledge. That is where the expert obtains his faith in this triad as the ideal of knowledge" (1979, 115). Epidemiologists want to be certain about risk, to be direct and clear in their communication of that risk, and they desire to create a vivid picture of events. However, as Callon and his colleagues point out, uncertainty does not lend itself to this type of certainty. When it comes to flu, one can be certain only about the continuation of uncertainty. The past is often used as a lens to project risk onto the future, however flawed this procedure might be. As Philip Alcabes quips, "Anxiety is no statistician" (2009, 222).

The problem boils down to this: Prior conceptualizations of a disease entity—such as the influenza virus—seep into modern-day scientific research programs and the collective thinking about that same disease agent.

As Fleck argues, "Concepts are not spontaneously created but are determined by their 'ancestors'" (1979, 20). In the case of the 2009 influenza pandemic, those ancestors were the 1918 H1N1 virus and the 1997, 2003, and 2005 H5N1 viruses. If, as scholars such as Philip Alcabes and Patricia Wald suggest, we are prone to crafting narratives about epidemics, then the stories we tell must also be familiar, or follow along a similar plot line. Even imagined, future outbreaks about deadly influenza must fit the mold in order to be intelligible (Alcabes 2009, Wald 2008).

As I have tried to show, the stories we create about pandemics are always unfinished. They loop back and forth in time and space and weave our fears about death and disease into the fabric of our daily uncertainties. Closing the gaps between reality and mythical tale, the Sirens' song of avian influenza draws us into a deeper dependency on global public health to keep us safe from harm. Or, if not to keep us entirely safe, then at least to alert us, to give us enough warning to protect ourselves. As Philip Alcabes suggests, in the modern age, we "appoint officials to do the imagining for us" (2009, 187), to peer into the abyss of disease and infection and predict what is coming. Epidemiologists become our "soothsayers" (2009, 186) or, to end this chapter where we began it, a collective modern Ulysses strapped to the mast of global public health. We want experts who are able to hear and heed the call of influenza so that they might know our future—and save us from it.

5

THE PREDICTABLE UNPREDICTABILITY
OF VIRUSES AND THE CONCEPT
OF "STRATEGIC UNCERTAINTY"

> Every outbreak is unique. Every new strain of virus is unique and until the
> outbreak has progressed you don't know what it's going to do and so it's a
> matter of making decisions with incomplete information.
>
> RICHARD BESSER, CDC Daily Press Briefing, April 2009

Gene Segment NP. Biological function: *The nucleoprotein (NP) gene of Influenza A plays a role in determining host specificity (which birds and/or mammals each strain of virus is capable of infecting). Although the segment is also
involved in viral replication, the NP protein is better known for its ability to interact with host proteins and to affect gene expression in the host.* Pathographic
function: *This chapter of the pathography continues our examination of the
biological, social, and political/economic narratives of influenza from the macro
level. The predictable unpredictability of viruses was utilized strategically by
scientists and epidemiologists alike to retain scientific authority during the 2009
pandemic. Here, uncertainty related to both the H1N1 virus and the "nature"
of the developing pandemic undergirded the call for further scientific research
on influenza as well as the construction of viral expertise itself.*

Uncertainty is a hot topic in the twenty-first century, much debated and
discussed in policy and academic circles, as well as in popular media. One
need only look to the ongoing global economic crisis, scientific research on

the effects of manmade climate change, or the 2011 Fukushima Daiichi nuclear disaster to see examples of "uncertainty" playing out in the so-called real world. Especially observable throughout the 2009 pandemic, uncertainty is as rife within global public health as it is in economic forecasting. The ostensibly new, or reinvigorated, concept of uncertainty remains as pervasive inside the World Health Organization as it is inside the International Monetary Fund or the World Bank. This type of omnipresent and sustained uncertainty, it seems, is now ubiquitous to modern life. Dealing with such extended and global crisis situations[1] has predicated a new type of public health response as well as need for a new type of analytic.

Through the months in which I worked closely with and spoke to various scientists and policymakers, the term uncertainty was rarely used in normal day-to-day conversations, during teleconferences, or in the various meetings I attended. However, the people around me often discussed information gaps, or what they didn't yet know, and the sheer unpredictability of the virus itself. In the many informal conversations between colleagues that I observed, the talk frequently turned to questions regarding the severity of the virus and its biological makeup and origins, the problems in obtaining crucial clinical information from affected areas, or about the difficulty of ascertaining the "denominator" of cases—how many individuals had been infected with the virus. There was much that was unknown about the emergent outbreak, and efforts were constantly being made to ascertain as much information as possible in order to lessen this uncertainty.

Uncertainty is, of course, nothing new within the realm of science—epidemiology and virology included. The scientific process was crafted, at least in part, to deal with the rather slippery reality of uncertainties in the world beyond the laboratory. Scholars in the field of science and technology studies have often focused on the ways in which uncertainty in science is artfully turned into scientific fact (see Callon 1999 [1986], Knorr-Cetina 1999, Latour and Woolgar 1979, Shapin and Schaffer 1985). Science produces facts and theories about the world through the practice of examining the realm of the unknown. Examinations of the daily practice of science have highlighted just how adept scientists are at utilizing the scientific method both to garner and to retain a certain authority in relationship to their subjects and fields. Indeed, I will argue throughout this chapter that scientific authority persists not despite uncertainty, but because of it. Uncertainty is the fertile ground for further scientific research and funding on influenza. Sustaining a partial uncertainty, grounded in the ontological unpredictability of viruses, and the effective management of that uncertainty through the production of scientific facts—or certainty— about the virus, helped professionals working in global public health to maintain the current research paradigm. It is this strategic utilization of uncertainty to positive effect that is the focus of my examination here.

In this line of thinking, then, one might make a valid point by arguing that an examination of uncertainty within public health is anything but new. Scholars of the themes of risk and preparedness have often pointed out how uncertainty is used within public health and policy circles to undergird planning and research paradigms to cope with possible future biological threats such as devastating pandemics (see Lakoff and Collier 2008). This type of uncertainty is conceptually related to a risk that occurs at some point in the future, but not to one that is unfurling in the present moment. I will argue below that the meaning of uncertainty itself has shifted. Uncertainty as it pertains to risk and preparedness for a *possible* infectious disease event differs qualitatively from uncertainty as it pertains to risk in the present moment or immediate future *during* an infectious disease event. There is little risk of undermining scientific authority when admitting that the future cannot be predicted (partially due to the fact that the specific infectious agent cannot be known in advance). Intuitively, one would surmise that there would be a much greater loss of authority as a result of admitting that the present moment was unpredictable because the disease agent itself, as well as the parameters of the developing situation, was not fully understood. This is why, in the not so distant past, public health professionals were often loath to openly discuss uncertainty. Throughout the early months of the 2009 H1N1 influenza pandemic, however, top public health officials regularly explained the uncertainty of the developing situation and appealed to the general public's understanding and patience. These pleas were often coupled with scientific explanations of the complex, ever-changing, and ambiguous situation, with the influenza virus itself being cast as "predictably unpredictable" in its biology, behavior, and spread. Public health professionals habitually and liberally used the concept of uncertainty in official communications to justify immediate response measures or to preempt and clarify any future changes in recommendations and actions. In effect, then, scientific authority was at least partially maintained through *a strategic deployment of biological uncertainty* regarding the H1N1 virus itself.

In what follows, I will first examine how biological science has effectively underpinned the rhetorical casting of the virus itself as innately "unpredictable." Analyzing scientific articles, media stories, quotes from top scientists and epidemiologists, and data gathered throughout my fieldwork, I will attempt to highlight how the influenza virus's predictable unpredictability—a term scientists and epidemiologists frequently used to describe the virus both in conversations with me and in the press (Altman 2009, Sepkowitz 2009)—is connected to the creation of a sustained uncertainty within influenza science. I then move on to look at how other "information gaps" are linked to uncertainty during an influenza outbreak, analyzing a random selection of media reports and interviews as well as relying on my own experience working within the CDC during the so-called second wave of the 2009 H1N1 pandemic. I argue that the fostering and public expression of scientific uncertainty was used strategically to either gain or retain trust during the 2009 H1N1 pandemic. The frequent deployment of what I will term "strategic uncertainty"[2] was, and largely remains, an effective method of retaining authority and control during an outbreak of infectious disease. Management of a sustained and partial ambiguity[3] or uncertainty in relationship to the production of scientific knowledge about the influenza virus itself becomes a tool for crafting and retaining scientific expertise throughout a crisis—with "strategic uncertainty" at the forefront of a new "epidemic order"[4] in global public health.

The Scientifically Predictable Unpredictability of Influenza

As soon as rumors and media reports regarding an unusual, late-season outbreak of influenza in Mexico began to circulate in March 2009, international scientists and epidemiologists working on influenza in public health focused upon a set of objectives that related to gaining a better understanding of the virus itself. First, public health agencies sought to obtain samples of the virus; next, virologists began to subtype those samples in order to ascertain which specific strain of influenza virus was causing the outbreaks; concurrently, evolutionary virologists began an immediate, international and collaborative effort to genetically sequence and analyze the virus in order to better understand its origins. As discussed in more depth in chapter 1 of this book, many public health experts believed that knowing more about the genetic makeup and origins of the influenza virus might help them to make better predictions not only about the severity and spread of the virus, but about the scope of the burgeoning pandemic. Thus, gathering information about the biology of the virus itself was crucial not only to the analysis of events as they unfolded in Mexico and in the southernmost states of the United States, but to the ability of public health experts to predict the immediate future.

By the end of April, it was evident to many of the virologists and epidemiologists who specialized in influenza that something big was unfurling. An influenza pandemic was at hand. The question then became, how bad would it be? At this stage, data regarding the severity of the H1N1 virus mattered. Severity, however, is not a concept that is easily defined, especially as it related to the 2009 H1N1 pandemic. Generically speaking, understanding severity involves knowing something about a virus's virulence and transmissibility, as well as being able to calculate the percentage of severe cases or deaths out of the total number of persons infected. Information that pertained to severity was hard to come by, especially in the first weeks of the pandemic, and people I spoke with often complained about the absence of "good data" on the total number of infections. The "problem of the denominator" and of better data regarding the biological attributes of the virus itself were often cast in the conversations I had with public health experts about the early days of the pandemic as the key pieces of information that epidemiologists needed in order to recommend an appropriate set of responses and often chronically lacked. One of the biggest problems seemed to be the "unpredictability" of the virus. This rather predictable unpredictability would become central to the story that was developing about the 2009 H1N1 pandemic.

In an analysis of the characteristic stories or narratives constructed about infectious disease outbreaks, scholar Priscilla Wald has suggested that "As epidemiologists trace the routes of microbes, they catalog the spaces and interactions of global modernity." Going further, she adds that "the outbreak narrative is itself like the epidemiological map and the electron microscope, a tool for making the invisible appear; it borrows, it attests to, and helps to construct expertise." (Wald 2008, 2, 39.) Following Wald's lead, then, I argue that it is necessary to read closely and begin to critically examine the narratives about unpredictability and uncertainty at the heart of the 2009 H1N1 pandemic. By doing so, we can begin to unpack how the representation of the virus as unpredictable was strategically utilized—operating at least in part as a rhetorical tool—to maintain scientific authority throughout the pandemic.

From the start, uncertainty about the virus was rife.[5] Some of the first media articles published about the outbreak highlight how the virus itself was being cast as intrinsically unpredictable. One of the earliest stories on the pandemic in *Science* suggested that "Much confusion surrounds the origins of the virus, why it seems to cause severe disease in Mexico and not elsewhere, and the overall threat it poses to the world. 'Right now, there's more unknown than there is known,' says microbiologist Francis Plummer." This particular article, first published on May 1, goes on to quote then–acting CDC Director Richard Besser as attesting to the fact that decisions were being made based on "incomplete information." (Cohen and Enserink 2009a, 572, 573.) The very next week, *Science* again reported that although information was being collected and shared internationally—and at unprecedented speed—there continued to be many "mysteries" about the virus (Cohen 2009b, 701). A segment on the developing situation first broadcast on May 1 and then published on NPR reported that "Experts still lack critical information about the virus" (Silberner and Greenfieldboyce 2009). An article in the *New York Times* during the first week of the outbreak emphasized the fact that even the WHO had admitted uncertainty about the virus, stating that "The World Health Organization said over the weekend that the new swine flu virus had the potential to cause another pandemic, but that it had no way of knowing whether it actually would." Within the same article, the virus itself was being blamed for the uncertainty, while the authority of the scientists was upheld. The writer explained that "For all that scientists have learned about influenza since the catastrophic pandemic of 1917–19, one thing has not changed: the predictably unpredictable nature of the viruses that cause it." (Altman 2009.)

The virus in these narratives is often described as a "mystery"—the implication being that unpredictability is an ontological property of the virus itself. That unpredictability, in turn, leads to an operative condition of "uncertainty" for public health. It is not inconsequential that the situation with influenza is consistently cast as inherently unpredictable; there is no end to uncertainty in this formulation. Indeed, there is also no clear beginning, as the virus is consistently put in a comparative frame with other pandemic influenzas viruses from the past. A scientific article published online in *Science* on May 11 stated that "although substantial uncertainty remains, clinical severity appears less than that seen in the 1918 influenza pandemic but comparable with that seen in the 1957 pandemic." Here, scientists have begun to analyze the "uncertainty" of the 2009 H1N1 virus in relationship to other viruses with the same or greater amount of "unpredictability." The scientists collectively argue that "There are uncertainties about all aspects of this outbreak, including the virulence, transmissibility, and origin of the virus, and this in turn results in uncertainty in judging the pandemic potential of the virus and when reactive public health responses, such as recommendations to stay at home or to close schools, should be implemented in individual countries." Uncertainty is mentioned no less than five times throughout the text of the article, but the writers still voice confidence that "uncertainty should diminish rapidly in coming weeks as more data on severe cases in the United States and other countries becomes available." (Fraser et al. 2009, 1557, 1560.)

By the end of May, two months after the beginning of the pandemic, statements about the unpredictability of the virus by and among scientists were already legion. *Science* reported that data on the virus remained "fuzzy" and quoted a prominent epidemiologist saying that "There's nothing more predictable about flu than its unpredictability." In the same article, Robert Webster was quoted as declaring that "You can't lay down rules for flu viruses—they'll break them every time. It's almost as though the virus reads them and says, 'I'll do the damn opposite'" (Cohen and Enserink 2009c, 997, 996). As Ann Schuchat of the CDC stated: "We're at early days in understanding this virus. . . . It is early days, and with influenza, we always want to be humble and know that things can change and it can be unpredictable" (Silberner and Greenfieldboyce 2009).

A little less than a year later, by late February 2010, the public consensus seemed to be that the pandemic was all but over. Infection rates were low and a second wave had never really materialized. Hundreds of thousands of vaccines the world over were left unused. But even so, uncertainty regarding the virus and the H1N1 outbreak not only lingered in the scientific realm, it seemed to be actively promoted. Reporting on a news teleconference, a HealthDay article quoted several top epidemiologists as warning against a too easy "dismissal" of H1N1, or having a "false sense of security." A professor of public health argued during the conference that " 'The flu is very hard to predict and what you think you know is only what happened before. There can always be a surprise' " (Gardner 2010). *Science* called H1N1 the "virus of the year" and suggested that it would "go down in history more for causing confusion than catastrophe" (Cohen and Enserink 2009b). And Carl Zimmer, a prominent science writer, wrote in his blog for *Discover* magazine that the flu strain was "nothing if not surprising," both in the form of its emergence and by virtue of the fact that by February 2010—the middle of the traditional flu season in the northern hemisphere—H1N1 had "dwindled away to very low levels and stayed there." In other words, the virus was unpredictable not only for its makeup and its severity, but for the pattern of its spread and disappearance. Zimmer argued that the virus "continues to move enigmatically ahead of our understanding." (Zimmer 2010.)

Of course, scientists and public health experts are not only accustomed to coping with the various difficulties in dealing with uncertainty, but well-versed in the more overt strategic and political uses of uncertainty as a device for the retention of authority. In an article on uncertainty published in the *American Journal of Public Health* in 2005, the co-authors working in public health stressed that "In our current regulatory system, debate over science has become a substitute for debate over policy" (Michaels and Monforton 2005, S45). The focus of the article is the use of uncertainty by defendants in environmental health lawsuits and public hearings, but the issues discussed in relation to the environmental arena can also shed light on similar types of arguments and debates regarding infectious disease (debates over vaccine safety or the charge of undue influence within the WHO being pertinent examples). The authors acknowledge that while much of public health policy is grounded in uncertainty, public health practitioners must recognize that fact while still using the "best evidence available" for their decision-making.

The WHO itself used the defense of uncertainty in responding to a charge in the *British Medical Journal* that it had exaggerated the threat from the H1N1 virus as a result of conflicts of interest involving some of its scientific advisers who had connections with the pharmaceuticals industry.[6] The WHO declared that "influenza viruses are unstable and can undergo rapid and significant mutations, making it difficult to predict whether the moderate impact would be sustained. This uncertainty, which persuaded WHO and many national health authorities to err on the side of caution, was further enforced by the behavior of past pandemics, which varied in their severity during first and second waves of international spread" (World Health Organization 2010). In its response to its critics, the WHO not only discussed its evidence and data, but openly admitted the underlying biological uncertainty of the virus itself. This adept rhetorical move distanced the organization from the source of the uncertainty, instead locating it within the realm of nature or biology. More research on the virus would therefore be required in order to better understand the severity of influenza outbreaks in the future. The scientific authority of the WHO was thus kept intact, even in the face of a sustained uncertainty.

In part, these "strategic" deployments of uncertainty work because the uncertainty is often displaced onto "nature" or "society" (Shackley and Wynne 1996)—entities such as the virus itself or the general public—both perceived as inherently out of the control of the laboratory or field epidemiologist. Trevor Pinch's seminal work on certainty in solar neutrino science (1981) showed how scientists often pointed to other disciplines or fields in which work was being done on the same problem as the source of uncertainty. The scientists' confidence in their own work or discipline remained unshaken. In the case of virologists, epidemiologists, and other public health experts during the 2009 H1N1 pandemic, uncertainty was primarily displaced upon the virus itself, with the virus being cast as biologically unpredictable. This unpredictability works, however, because unpredictability in the case of influenza is ultimately predictable. Thus, the creation of certainty about uncertainty becomes an effective method of retaining scientific authority during the pandemic.

Expanding Uncertainty

Much of the language used in the section above by public health professionals to describe the influenza virus during press interviews focused on terms such as "uncertainty" and "unpredictability," but a more generic uncertainty was also revealed in relationship to other "information gaps." Scientists and public health officials often privately grappled with what they viewed as a constantly changing and largely ambiguous situation. In the private meetings or conversations that I observed, public health experts often used phrases such as "we think" or "it seems" rather than "we know" or "it is" to reflect their own doubts about the type and quality of the information they had access to or were deriving from the various graphs, tables, charts, maps, and case counts that were in circulation throughout the 2009 H1N1 pandemic. Although much of the doubt remained centered on the "biology of the bug," uncertainty quickly expanded to include other aspects of the pandemic.

While working within the CDC in the fall of 2009, I attended several meetings or teleconferences that pertained to the 2009 H1N1 pandemic. By October, the experts whom I worked with were feeling the full effects of the "damned if they do, damned if they don't" paradox within public health (Altman 2009)—the precariousness of either sounding a false alarm or underreacting in the wake of the discovery of a novel and widely circulating influenza virus. The key to certainty during a pandemic is accurate information—data that epidemiologists everywhere lamented they were lacking, especially during the early weeks of the pandemic. Information was being circulated in a transparent manner. In fact, many public health experts felt that they were "drowning" in data, but that little of it was "actionable" or usable (more on this in the following chapter). By using the term "actionable," public health experts were expressing their frustration that official case counts and other "numbers" being shared did not provide any clarity on the overall situation. At stake was the ability to predict the immediate future and issue recommendations for action.

In interviews with public health experts during the latter stages of the 2009 H1N1 pandemic, I often brought up the topic of uncertainty in relationship to information gaps and risk in order to understand—in more specificity—what public health experts meant when they utilized the term. These conversations often shed much-needed light on how uncertainty was deployed, both in a general sense and in the bounded realm of influenza research and prevention. I discovered that there was a disparity between what people working in public health meant by the term and how uncertainty was perceived in the popular media or the general public. The tension between understanding uncertainty and the ability to make predictions during an outbreak was often highlighted. During discussions about uncertainty, public health experts frequently described what they saw as essential to understanding the unpredictability of an outbreak of influenza. These conversations did not necessarily center around the unpredictability of the virus—although that never really disappeared as a concern—but around the comprehension of risk vis-à-vis the inbuilt unpredictability of an influenza pandemic. In essence, the public health experts I spoke with told me time and time again that there would never be "certainty" during an outbreak of influenza, no matter how much they knew about the virus or the current situation.

The following excerpt from one of my interviews reveals the underlying problem with using objective data to make predictions during a pandemic:

TM: I'm not sure I understand uncertainty. And I don't think I understand probability and risk.

Ben Cowling: Well, even scientists really don't understand risk. (*Laughter.*)

TM: Statistics are a hard thing . . . I mean, intellectually, they are easy to understand, but they are not an easy thing to apply.

BC: That's right, that's right. And uncertainty is the real big one, because, you know, whenever you see the media reporting numbers, it's just "numbers as truth." But actually there's always a lot of uncertainty about what numbers really mean. When they go up and down, people would like to have a lot of interpretation about why they go up or down. But quite often, it can be random variation.

What becomes important here is the *understanding* of the "numbers," the various epidemiological data as they relate to uncertainty, risk, and the ability of public health professionals to predict the immediate future during a pandemic. Numbers here are not as "objective" as one might first conjecture, despite the fact that they are the lingua franca of epidemiological science. If these numbers ultimately form the basis for many of the decisions being made during a pandemic, then what does it mean when the public health experts themselves admit that the data are themselves imbued with a certain amount of uncertainty? Uncertainty here is prepackaged in; it adheres to the data.

Internationally recognized virologist Gavin Smith cautioned me about the dangers of using such information to make predictions about how a pandemic might unfold. As he explained to me: "You can look into the past, but you can't look at the future. To make a prediction about the future, you've got to get the virus, put it into a ferret or some other animal model, see if it kills them, look at how many . . . look at mortality and what virulence and what transmissibility and then you can make some sort of prediction." Again, uncertainty about the course of a pandemic is rhetorically tied to the actions of the virus itself. The virus here needs to be observed directly in order to know something about how it works. The past only provides a guide for what may happen during the present, but can never predict the future. Everything here is about *comparison*—either with the past or with other locations during the same time period. Without comparison, there can be no sense-making in the present tense.

A chronic lack of comparative data—just think of the debate over the number of fatalities compared with the total number of cases, referred to as the "denominator debate"—often leads to confusion about the immediate future and a continuation of uncertainty. As Dr. Thomas Tsang explained it to me: "We always talk about objective evidence and objective data. In the real world, they don't come in handy. There's always going to be important data gaps, knowledge gaps, even interpretation gaps. So it's never a perfect situation in which to make decisions." In a real sense, Dr. Tsang's remark uncovers the construction of a type of *sustained* uncertainty within public health in relationship to infectious disease outbreaks. No matter how much data (quantity) or how "objective" the data (quality), there will always be a "subjective" (interpretation) gap that leads to uncertainty during an outbreak. When I asked if this type of uncertainty would be repeated—ad infinitum—into the future, Dr. Tsang responded that it *certainly* would. Thus, information not only about the influenza virus, but other epidemiological data produced during an outbreak, simply feeds back into the uncertainty loop.

In response to the criticisms from the *British Medical Journal* in June 2010, the WHO rejected wholesale the idea that the pandemic had been "hyped" in collusion with vaccine manufacturers. In its briefing note released on June 10, the WHO reiterated the evidence-based claim that severity of an influenza outbreak is variable—and can change in regard to time, place and population. At first glance, the briefing looks like a typical case of post hoc fact formation, with the WHO presenting documentation to bolster its case. Looking more carefully, however, one can see evidence of strategic uncertainty being expertly deployed. Severity is difficult to pin down because it requires a case-by-case *interpretation* of the data. It is the formulation of uncertainty as part of the permanent process of public health that interests me. How has uncertainty become one of the key components of global public health's rationale for its response to the 2009 H1N1 pandemic? More importantly, what does this collective turn toward, or partial embracing of uncertainty signal?

Strategic Uncertainty and Scientific Authority

By the end of 2009, little uncertainty was still being expressed—either publicly or privately—concerning the duration, severity, or overall course of the H1N1 pandemic. The 2009 H1N1 pandemic had, by all accounts, turned out to be similar in severity to that of a normal or "mild" flu season. Facts were known; a collective sense of scientific certainty regarding certain aspects of the pandemic—about the biological makeup of the virus, its severity and potential duration, and the immediate risk it posed to society—had all but resumed. Many of the scientists and epidemiologists that I interviewed as late as May 2010, however, expressed a continued uncertainty relating to the H1N1 virus itself. From a virology standpoint, some public health experts worried openly that there might be an antigenic shift or a recombination event that could transform the H1N1 virus into something more ominous. In conversations throughout the latter stages of the pandemic, public health experts consistently used this uncertainty— the predicable unpredictability of the influenza virus—to support not only their past and future decisions, but their present actions as well. In what follows, I will use the CDC's and the WHO's deployment of uncertainty about the H1N1 virus during different phases of the pandemic to suggest that a new type of strategic uncertainty was being used within global public health as an effective rhetorical tool to retain scientific authority *during* this infectious disease event.

From the very beginning of the pandemic in April, CDC officials began to communicate uncertainty about the situation (see first section above). The then–acting director of the CDC, Richard Besser, stated that the agency's overall objective during the event had been to "tell everything we knew, everything we didn't know and what we were doing to get the answers." In an article on the crisis communication style of Richard Besser, the journal *Nature* praised Besser's management of the situation, noting how Besser's overt use of uncertainty helped to shape the tenor of the entire US response. The article quotes several prominent members of the international public health community as attesting to Besser's overall skill in "communicating uncertainty." Even noted expert on the 1976 influenza pandemic, Harvey Fineberg, argued that the CDC's communication of uncertainty during the pandemic under Besser was exemplary. Although the *Nature* article also argued that Besser had miscalculated the "political ramifications" of the CDC's more aggressive early actions (such as recommendations on school closures), the fact that Besser himself was able to parlay his communication of uncertainty into several lucrative job offers should be seen as objective evidence that his strategic use of uncertainty was effective. In his subsequent job as the health analyst for *Good Morning America* on ABC, Besser "still projects uncertainty." (Maher 2010, 150–52.)

My own interviews with public health experts outside of the United States support this view of the CDC's handling of the pandemic. The CDC was rarely overtly criticized. Instead, the CDC's strategy of "saying what you don't know" had been actively replicated in other locations. Public relations experts have actively coached public health experts in the art of crisis communication, advocating honesty and transparency over the projection of absolute authority. In a conversation about the focus on uncertainty throughout the pandemic, scholar and former journalist Thomas Abraham suggested to me that the CDC—as the reigning "gold standard" of epidemiological science with a global reputation to match—had utilized the concept of uncertainty more often, and with greater impunity, than other national or international health agencies had dared. It is interesting to note here, then, that the CDC has not come under the same scrutiny or criticism as the WHO for its response to the pandemic.

Also at stake in the *British Medical Journal*'s 2010 article was the WHO's decision in May of 2009 to change its definition of a pandemic, striking a key phrase that had described a pandemic as an outbreak causing an "enormous" number of deaths. The authors of the article blamed, in part, the WHO's poor communication of risk, quoting one expert in risk communication as stating that "The problem is not so much that communicating uncertainty is difficult, but that uncertainty was not communicated" (Cohen and Carter 2010). Responding to criticisms that the WHO had "overreacted" and "inflated risk" during the early weeks of the outbreak, the United Nations influenza expert Keiji Fukuda argued that the pandemic was not over yet, and that the risk was "real" (UN News Centre 2010).

Uncertainty during an infectious disease outbreak is by its very nature undisciplined and anxiety-provoking. Uncertainty is not easily managed, either within the confines of a laboratory dealing with the virus or in the world at large coping with an outbreak. All of the various scientific and epidemiological graphs, tables, maps, and lists of numbers showing lab-confirmed H1N1 cases that were produced throughout the pandemic to track the peaks and valleys of the flu season were partial attempts by public health experts to alleviate some of the uncertainty surrounding the influenza virus itself. This creation and circulation of knowledge about the immediate or distant future—"anticipatory knowledge"—is an attempt to wield authority over uncertainty, to make the unpredictable more predictable, to "project" competence and power, to create order out of potential disorder (Nelson, Geltzer, and Hilgartner 2008). As scholars of the 2009 H1N1 pandemic have pointed out, both politicians and public health officials have opted for two rhetorical moves, often in the same sentence, that functioned both to sound an alarm and to reassure the public about epidemic events (Briggs and Nichter 2009, 191). In practice, the scientists must walk the fine line between under and overstating uncertainties in relationship to a politically-charged issue (Shackley and Wynne 1996, 278). Reports on the 2009 H1N1 pandemic constituted metapragmatic accounts (Briggs and Nichter 2009)—or accounts of the accounts—of how epidemiologists, clinicians, and others produced and circulated knowledge. Looking critically, then, at the narratives around the uncertainty of influenza, we can see that a certain type of "anticipatory uncertainty" is being deployed. Wald has argued that "the epidemiological narrative is, like the microscope, a technology" (2008, 19). The construction of sustained uncertainty—both now and in the immediate future—provides scientists with a certain flexibility, a maneuverable bracketing of the future that is used to help control the present moment, a narrative tool for both gaining and retaining scientific authority during an outbreak of infectious disease. What cannot be known *now* can be further researched, it can be known *later*. In this deft move, a certain amount of biological uncertainty does not trouble scientific authority, but helps to further generate it.

In an article looking at uncertainty in relationship to climate science and environmental policy, Shackley and Wynne suggested that uncertainty has its uses, especially for scientists; it acts as an "alibi," a way to support further research funding, and as a hedge against the "encroachment" of policymakers into their realm of expertise. Uncertainty is negotiated in the semipublic interactions among scientists, policymakers, and politicians (1996, 277). Brian Campbell has argued that the very existence of uncertainty is evidence of "continual interpretation and negotiation," and that scientists who are asked to perform the role of expert in public hearings commonly "state that there is uncertainty, and that this type of argument can be managed and accepted as authoritative". According to Campbell, this "maneuvering in relation to uncertainty demonstrates a *strategic* importance of the issue of uncertainty to expert arguments." I take his use of "strategic" seriously, as well as the suggestion that the strategic use of uncertainty reveals the politics inherent in policy science. For Campbell, uncertainty is not the cause of policy debates, but their result. Uncertainty is a *flexible tool* that aids in negotiation of authority. (Campbell 1985, 430, 431, 445, 447.) The 2009 H1N1 pandemic might be seen as a "boundary-ordering device" (Shackley and Wynne 1996, 280), where uncertainty helps to redefine the authority of both scientists and epidemiologists. In essence, the strategic use of uncertainty allows the construction of a type of "certainty *about* uncertainty." In turn, policymakers can use uncertainty in a strategic way to "deflect unwelcome attention and criticism of the policy process." All of this does nothing to undermine the authority of science. Indeed, the strategic use of uncertainty strengthens that authority. Science is once again seen as the only way of closing a critical "information gap," and the authority of the current scientific paradigm further strengthens the reigning "policy order." (Shackley and Wynne 1996, 281, 283, 287.)

Claiming that there is uncertainty is in no way an admission that the scientist is in no position to judge—quite the contrary (Campbell 1985, 449). In fact, the strategic deployment of uncertainty guarantees that scientific authority will be maintained, casting the scientist/epidemiologist as the only person qualified to judge an uncertain situation. Scientists know *better*, if they do not know *all*. They have the tools to know further, to gather more information. In essence, if uncertainty somehow necessitates a return to certainty, then the strategic use of uncertainty ensures that science will be the discipline asked to shepherd us back to more solid, or certain, ground. But as Campbell points out, the "problem" of uncertainty cannot be dealt with quantitatively; it is a "social" problem (1985, 450). It was the rhetorical trick of deploying uncertainty during the 2009 H1N1 pandemic that has so deftly maintained the need for more qualitative data to interpret the pandemic.

Science and technology studies scholar Susan Leigh Star has studied the ways in which "local uncertainties" are transformed into "global certainty", or facts. In Star's theory, belief is a core facet of the ability of working scientists to transform uncertainty into certainty. As Star points out at the beginning of her analysis, "scientists constantly face uncertainty" (1985, 392). This is, of course, no less true thirty years later than it was when Star first began to study uncertainty as a phenomenon. However, Star's article also reflects the sea change in scientists' relationship to uncertainty. Her work centers on how various types of uncertainty were completely elided from published scientific work through six mechanisms for creating global certainty: attributing certainty to other fields; maintaining that technical failures were to blame for any errors, rather than the internal processes of science; the creation of ideal types; shifting evaluation criteria to mask uncertainty; generalizing results in an ad hoc manner; and using internal debates or arguments over *how* to perform research to "subsume" uncertainty about *whether* to perform research. All of this "management of uncertainty" in the local setting had to "satisfy local constraints *and* create global certainty." (Star 1985, 407–12, 413.)

In effect, what Star argued in the 1980s was that local uncertainty formed the basis of global certainty about scientific facts and about the value of entire global research paradigms. This was one of the reasons why scientific theories could persist well into the future. The transformation of uncertainty into certainty was the most efficient tool for sustaining a scientific paradigm indefinitely. In 2010, however, the meaning of uncertainty itself has begun to shift. Uncertainty is no longer the "dirty secret" of science. To reflect this, I want to take Star's old argument and flip it to argue that *sustained uncertainty* is now what ultimately holds the global influenza research paradigm together. Strategic uncertainty does not necessarily need to be transformed into certainty in order for it to form the basis of a robust research paradigm. The CDC and WHO public responses to the 2009 H1N1 pandemic are examples of how effective the deployment of strategic uncertainty can be for the retention of authority during an outbreak of infectious disease.

Strategic Uncertainty and the Creation of Knowledge

Medical anthropologists and observers of global public health are rarely strangers to the deployment of strategic uncertainty. In recent editorials on the 2009 H1N1 pandemic, anthropologists have effectively argued that what biological and epidemiological approaches to infectious diseases lack is a social or cultural component (see Atlani-Duault and Kendall 2010, Singer 2009). These prominent scholars are not so much critiquing influenza science or global health response per se, but rather suggesting that their own area of expertise should be more efficiently utilized in order to fill up any critical gaps in data about how different socioeconomic groups or cultures cope with pandemics and devise and implement public health measures. They are arguing for inclusion in the larger scientific paradigm based on their own social-scientific authority, deploying the concept of uncertainty to strengthen the case for their own discipline's analysis of pandemics. Anthropology here is conceptualized as another effective tool for dealing with present and future uncertainty.

This chapter has been, in part, an attempt to ask a new kind of question about certainty and uncertainty within global public health. Can we be "certain" about "uncertainty"? How might uncertainty be sustained and utilized in relationship to the maintenance of scientific authority? Is this a new form of uncertainty or simply a new and more robust use of it? And, perhaps most importantly, how is the fuzzy line between biological "certainty" and "uncertainty" continuously renegotiated and/or maintained by the various scientists, epidemiologists, and other public health professionals working within public health?

Building out from Wittgenstein's last statements on certainty, the concepts of certainty and of knowledge are not all that different. Under Wittgenstein's formulation, certainty occurs the moment when someone "declares how things are." (1969, 3e, 6e). During the recent 2009 H1N1 influenza pandemic, public health experts declared vociferously and repeatedly that the situation was somehow fundamentally, naturally, biologically uncertain. Here I have attempted to examine how the meanings of words like "uncertainty" have shifted, how other concepts have changed along with them, and how they might then be used to craft a new type of epidemic order. If we take seriously Wittgenstein's postulate that "a meaning of a word is a kind of employment of it" (1969, 10e), then we must begin to further examine how the scientists and epidemiologists working in global public health utilize the term "uncertainty" in daily practice: what it might signify when it is used casually in relation to ongoing scientific work and attempts to gather epidemiological data; what it might signify when it is deployed within the public sphere; and, finally, how it might be utilized strategically vis-à-vis scientific authority.

This is not to argue, however, that present-day scientific authority rests solely upon the maintenance of uncertainty. Now, as ever, scientific expertise is firmly located in the ability to produce facts, or certainty, about the world in which we live. My goal in this chapter has been to point out how a new configuration of scientific authority within global public health straddles the ever-tenuous line between certainty and uncertainty, and to examine how biological uncertainty was deployed at key moments during an infectious disease outbreak to bolster that authority. As Wittgenstein pointed out before his death, one cannot begin to doubt without being certain, without first believing a set of propositions to be true. Thus, to translate Wittgenstein's propositions into the realm of public health, one cannot have biological uncertainty about a particular virus without first having created a baseline of scientific knowledge about an entire class of influenza viruses. Similar to the role of "failure" in perpetuating the need for further initiatives and programs within the development industry in Africa (Ferguson 1994), sustained uncertainty regarding the biological properties and characteristics of the H1N1 virus and its strategic deployment merely presupposes the need for the creation of further biological knowledge about the virus. This is how the trick works, and why the admission of uncertainty is no hindrance to the retention of authority in science or in global public health. In essence, we cannot produce knowledge about influenza without uncertainty.

Uncertainty and Information

The 2009 H1N1 pandemic constituted an event in which the infrastructures that undergird much of the day-to-day operations of global public health showed signs of strain. Overloaded with information and bogged down in response duties, epidemiologists and virologists everywhere were suddenly aware of the gaps and the friction—the uncertainty—inherent in global public health information and communication systems. These all too public problems had an ancillary benefit; the system under stress had the effect of making some of the more "invisible" beliefs and practices of epidemiologists and scientists "visible" even to an uninitiated observer (such as myself). Bowker and Star argue that "One cannot directly see relations such as membership, learning, ignoring, or categorizing." What one can see, however, especially during uncertain or stressful events when responsibilities need to be renegotiated, are boundary infrastructures or "objects that cross larger levels of scale than boundary objects." (Bowker and Star 1999, 285, 287.) Epidemiological and scientific information related to the 2009 H1N1 pandemic was one such boundary infrastructure.

In the next chapter, I explore the concepts of certainty and uncertainty in relationship to information in public health through the lens of the 2009 H1N1 pandemic, beginning with an exploration of the ever-expanding definition of information in the twenty-first century. Relying on participant observation and data on information-sharing collected during the so-called second wave of the pandemic, I examine the various social, political, and cultural aspects of the generation and circulation of epidemiological information. Public health professionals often stressed a reliance on informal personal relationships to fill in any information gaps in more official sources or networks. Successful past efforts to increase transparency and information flow in public health accidentally created what many in the field refer to as a "data deluge," and has also highlighted a significant new obstacle—that of getting access to the "context" deemed crucial to any decision-making process. The next chapter explores what global health experts mean when they use the term "context," and suggests that the problem of the data deluge does not center on the creation of more or better information or technology, but in understanding how communication and personal interactions shape the production of "good" or "actionable" information.

6

THE ANTHROPOLOGY OF
GOOD INFORMATION

Data Deluge, Knowledge, and Context
in Global Public Health

There's a thin line between how much you need to know and what you
want to know.

An epidemiologist on the ever-present need for information, July 2009

As the confidence men put it, the good sucker always wants the best of it
[information].

HAROLD GARFINKEL, *Toward a Sociological Theory of Information*

Gene Segment NA. Biological function: *The neuraminidase (NA) enzyme has
several functions at different stages of the viral replication cycle. The most important of these are the early stages of cell infection and the last stages of release
and spread of progeny virions from the host cell. Due to its role in influenza's
transmissibility and ability to infect the ciliated epithelium of human airways,
neuraminidase is a target of antiviral drugs developed to inhibit viral function.
The NA gene segment is closely monitored for any changes in its genetic makeup.*
Pathographic function: *This chapter of the pathography examines the "life
cycle" of information in public health from an ethnographic and sociological perspective. The effective and timely exchange of "good" information is seen as the
lifeblood of global public health. The process of turning data into information,
and then turning so-called good information into "actionable" knowledge to inform response activities, relies upon experts to use their own personal and collective institutional experience—or "context"—to analyze and interpret circulating
information. Context here is integral not only to the construction and maintenance of the global health network, but also to the formation of expertise itself.*

Walking down the halls of the Centers for Disease Control in the fall of 2009, I quickly became recognizable as the "Berkeley person" doing research on information-sharing and sense-making during infectious disease outbreaks. Two weeks into my tenure, I started being hailed by my academic association and playfully taunted with echoes of my research question: "Hey, Berkeley! Have you figured out the problem of information yet?"

The joke belied the fact that people were often extremely eager to talk with me about the various issues associated with information in public health: gathering data, getting access to various types of data and information, deciphering information in the form of graphs or tables or numbers, generating and recirculating information, and discerning what was often referred to as any "actionable" or "good" information that might be used to help halt the spread of a growing pandemic. When I explained my research goals, people would often let out an audible sigh expressing a type of "information fatigue"—a mental and sometimes physical exhaustion brought on by dealing with the daily glut of information. The public health professionals I knew well or interviewed in the United States and in Hong Kong habitually referred to the steady stream of emails, phone calls, meetings, and teleconferences as part of a "sea of information" or a veritable "data deluge." Already taxed with their regular duties of disease surveillance, prevention efforts, and outbreak response, public health workers everywhere felt that their burdens had exponentially increased throughout the first ten months of the 2009 H1N1 pandemic.

People regularly complained about "drowning" in information, about being bowled over by a never-ending series of "waves" of data, about having "barely a drop" of usable information in the oceans that crossed their desks each day. I rapidly discovered that the collective goal wasn't necessarily to become adept swimmers; rather, it seemed to be to simply tread water in the midst of a virtual sea of information. Throughout the year-long pandemic, experts continuously voiced a common longing for a more permanent solution to the problem of too much information, for a method or practice or tool that might help them cope with the overflow produced by rapidly improving technological systems of data generation and information-sharing. In the twenty-first century, in public health as in other realms that rely heavily upon digital information such as finance (Ho 2009) or journalism (Boyer 2013),[1] the primary problem is no longer necessarily getting access to information, but of effectively coping with an overabundance of it.

Prior experience with outbreaks of infectious diseases such as SARS and avian influenza had led to an increased global awareness of the problems in public health centered on obtaining timely access to accurate information. During the 2009 H1N1 pandemic, I could barely get through an entire conversation without someone directly linking SARS or avian influenza to the present-day problems of information. Post-SARS, it had become apparent to those within the global public health community that information on infectious disease outbreaks of global importance needed to be: (1) verifiable from a trusted or validated source; (2) more appropriately disseminated; and (3) shared at a faster rate. The public health community's subsequent emphasis on fostering greater transparency and information-sharing in public health, spearheaded by changes to the WHO's system for reporting infectious diseases, including the revision in 2005 of the International Health Regulations, solved some of the concerns over access to information, yet at the same time added an increased pressure to more quickly report validated—or good—information. After IHR revisions, the modern myth that increased transparency and access to more information would produce better information had been born. Yet, years after the world's first influenza pandemic in decades, it has become increasingly apparent to everyone working in public health that more information is not, in fact, necessarily better information. And while Big Data is now regularly touted as a solution to complex problems, the reality of information-sharing during the 2009 H1N1 pandemic highlighted other, more social—and pernicious—problems tied to the quality of the information being so readily shared.

This chapter examines how information in global public health networks is produced, managed, understood, and circulated during an outbreak. Using the 2009 H1N1 pandemic as a specific case study for examining the social practice and politics of information-sharing, I argue that informal networks—consisting of personal relationships—are crucial to the process of sharing sensitive, unvalidated, or what people called "good" information. The recent drive to foster greater efficiency in information-sharing created various technological, scientific, and institutional temptations to decontextualize information in order to share it more quickly. The end result was a problem of quality, not quantity. In this way, the largely political push toward greater transparency and faster information-sharing in public health aggravated a need for what the people I worked with often called "context."

As a concept used by public health professionals, "context" refers to the fusion of clinical and personal experience and intuition about a disease outbreak. To them, context is the key to transforming uncertainty into certainty, involving the human relationships and daily practices and experiences at the heart of both the production and the understanding of epidemiological information. If information is more about the production and circulation of data or facts, then context is more the circulation of experience and beliefs. As one expert explained it to me, context is what a person *really* knows. In other words, it is the creative synthesis of personal knowledge and impersonal data. Without context, facts (or the type of validated information that epidemiologists and scientists traffic in) are still viewed with a certain suspicion as to their soundness or applicability. Contextual information is the alchemical force that helps to turn information into knowledge or "good information."

Without its attendant context, information produced and circulated during the pandemic was deemed mostly, if not entirely, useless. Borrowing from sociologist Harold Garfinkel (2008), I argue that epidemiologists know the thing "good information" only through its usage or its usability. The problem of context in relationship to the analysis of information in global public health is focused on the perceived level of transparency about *the process or practice of analyzing information.* Throughout the 2009 pandemic, the thing that people most wanted to acquire, what they spent the largest amount of their time trying to gain access to, was not more information about case counts, or symptoms, or even about virulence, but information about how people were aggregating, analyzing, and producing information about the outbreak. In essence, the public health experts I knew were desperate to better understand their peers' thinking processes. They believed that this type of contextual information would help them to better decide which pieces of generic information—or aggregated data—about the outbreak were most important. In sum, they wanted context to help them separate out important signals from the collective noise.

The Data Deluge, or, Too Much of a Good Thing

On any given normal or "routine" day, an epidemiologist or analyst working within the framework of global public health can receive upward of three hundred email, text, and phone messages. During a severe outbreak of any disease of international importance,[2] or during a pandemic such as the 2009 H1N1 influenza, that daily number can reach as high as five hundred messages or more. Most public health experts also attend multiple daily and weekly team meetings—either in person within their own agencies, or virtually in the case of international meetings or meetings across agencies. This type of frenetic communications activity is a mechanism for both the production and sharing of the critical epidemiological information deemed so necessary for responding to the threat of any outbreak of infectious disease.

In this section, I examine a few select, but representative, conversations that took place during my observations and interviews in the fall of 2009 and spring of 2010, throughout what was generally referred to as the "second wave" of the 2009 H1N1 influenza pandemic. The discussions excerpted and analyzed below focus on the personal experiences of scientists, epidemiologists, and officials working inside the highly charged atmosphere of national public health agencies in the United States and in Hong Kong. As such, I take them to be demonstrative of the problems and practices of public health professionals working under the rubric of "global public health." The following examples are thus indicative of a particular type of political sensitivity. National public health agencies are often the clearing houses for local, national, and international information about outbreaks. People who work within the confines of national health policy inside large governmental agencies need to abide by strict protocols of information-sharing amidst their larger efforts to collect enough "good" information on which to base response recommendations. In examining here how public health professionals spoke about information, I am less attentive to the different types of specific information being discussed (clinical, laboratory, epidemiological, or contextual data), than I am to the similarities in the narratives of needing to cope with "too much" information.

I first began to hear about this data deluge while working at the CDC's Global Disease Detection and Operations Center (GDDOC) in the fall of 2009. In the elevator of Building 21, the building that houses the CDC's main Emergency Operations Center, I met a friendly man who was part of a special task force associated with the H1N1 response. After I explained my research, we briefly discussed how people made sense of all the information that they received on any given day. From his own direct experience, he said, there was entirely too much information for individuals to manage. People did their best, but he added that "It's getting to the point where it's 'information overload,' you know? It's hard to deal with everything that is coming at us."

While at the CDC, I spent a good deal of my free time discussing what it was like to work inside what is one of the seminal public health institutions in the world. One of the oldest and most experienced analysts in the GDDOC, Myron Schultz—or Mike—had an extensive, decades-long history in epidemiology. He had been trained under Alexander Langmuir as part of the Epidemiological Intelligence Service at the CDC and was a highly respected member of the analyst team, in no small part due to his wealth of personal knowledge and past experience. When I asked Mike about his job as an analyst working within global health, he said he had felt completely disoriented when he first started the job. Overwhelmed by the amount of information coming into the group mailbox, he recalled his initial desire to discover what the specific role of a global public health analyst was. Although Mike had decades of experience, he had been unsettled by the sheer workload and stress of being on the analyst team.

Mike's colleague, Rohit Chitale, on the other hand, found the work exhilarating. Rohit explained that only "adrenaline junkies" endure this kind of work within public health. Though decades younger than Mike, Rohit had been in the unit since its advent in 2006 and acted as the GDDOC's senior analyst. The parent program (Global Disease Detection) itself had been instituted in the wake of SARS, with the ever-present specter of a SARS-like disease or a deadly bird flu pandemic shrouding the future of public health. The GDDOC had been set up as part of the CDC's surveillance and response system specifically to focus on non-US or "global" disease events. Analysts received information and reports on disease outbreaks from all over the world, so the team was also an important part of the effort to help coordinate "global" or international responses to serious disease threats everywhere.

Kira Christian, the youngest and least senior analyst, agreed that analysts had to cope with a "deluge of emails." Her use of the phrase was coupled with the suggestion that it was easy to lose track of key information in the surge coming into the center on a day-to-day basis. All the analysts persistently expressed feelings of being overwhelmed by their email accounts, especially the constant stream of disease outbreak alerts from surveillance services. They regularly described the situation as "being inundated" or feeling "overloaded" by information. The feelings weren't new, however. The 2009 H1N1 pandemic had merely intensified both the situation and the sense of being overwhelmed by information. As just one example, at the height of the pandemic response, the CDC had over fifteen hundred individuals listed as active participants in response activities. By any measure, that is a vast amount of people sharing and generating information, all needing to be kept in the same informational loop.

During a private conversation in the office, Rohit explained to me that even in nonpandemic situations, he still received hundreds of emails in a day. I asked him to see how many he had already received that day. He walked over to his workstation, pulled up his inbox on one of his two monitor screens, and laughed out loud.

"It's only noon, and I have 244 mostly unread emails."

I asked him to break them down for me. Some had been sent directly to him, but most were addressed to the group outbreak mailbox, which autoforwarded messages into all staff inboxes. All work-related emails concerned two types of work. All the various reports that were automatically fed into his box Rohit labeled as "passive work." Whenever he or one of the other analysts had to go to a website or get information on an outbreak from someone in their network, that was "active work."

"The less active work I have to do, the better," he explained. In part, this was because looking for information could take up valuable hours better spent doing an analysis of all the information on an outbreak that the team had already received passively.

A lot of what the center did, Rohit said, was to field questions from people who "can't put things into context for themselves. People throw balls at us, and we have to get the answers, package them up, and hit them back to people."

The "balls" were all the discrete pieces of information that had to be stitched together and analyzed by the team before they could be "hit back"—or recirculated as more meaningful accretions or "chunks" of information. One of the core reasons articulated for the GDDOC's existence is, in part, to give other experts working within the CDC (or its partner agencies) the "context" they need in order to make informed decisions about outbreak response. In essence, Kira, Mike, and Rohit recontextualized all the decontextualized data that was circulated via the various surveillance and information-sharing networks.

From Rohit's perspective, there were two reasons for keeping on top of the data deluge. First, the job of an information analyst was to provide an overview of any given situation, or what epidemiologists call "situational awareness." Second, keeping abreast of all the information allowed public health professionals to better respond to outbreaks. Rohit conceptualized the essence of his job as "risk interpretation," and gave me a fictitious example to illustrate his meaning. He explained that the real difference between "getting information" and "getting verification" out of former communist and communist countries was that while you might get information out of a country like China, you would get little confirmation of that information. Because of this, and as the senior analyst, Rohit cautioned against over- or underestimating a disease threat based on "incomplete information." The team's directive in such a situation was to "Stay away from numbers, unless you've got a credible source." The task of locating credible or "good" information has become much more difficult, however, as the quantity of information has grown.

In many ways, the effect of the data deluge in public health mirrors a similar problem with data in genomics or any other technology-based science—a bottleneck effect occurs in any effort to churn out meaningful information from a glut of data constantly being fed into a system. What is required is less information, not more. Or, to phrase it more accurately, more selective information. More information has merely served to increase the level of complexity that analysts and others working in global public health need to cope with in daily practice. The technological capacity to produce and store large amounts information is, as some information scholars have argued, outstripping our human ability to process it. We are now living in the "zettabyte era" of "exafloods"—or as information scholar Luciano Floridi describes it, a "tsunami of bytes that is submerging the world" (2010, 6). Is it any wonder, then, that those working in public health are feeling the strain of this flood of information? The resultant data deluge in public health has led to a kind of communal nostalgia for the past, a time when there were far fewer epidemiologists involved in decision-making processes and response groups were small enough to have intimate knowledge of each other. This nostalgia flourishes, in part, because everyone knows that the "old" way of doing epidemiology is gone forever. In its wake is a new system of technologies, networks, and hierarchies of information-sharing that all contribute to an ever-growing glut of information—one most recently highlighted by the interest in and advancement of Big Data in the sciences.

At a conference held at Berkeley to discuss the 2009 H1N1 pandemic response, one local state public health worker summed up the problem of the data deluge with a metaphor: "There are so many facets of an outbreak, and there's no way to pool everything together. You have your data, they have theirs. It's like the Indian looking at the elephant—you have the trunk, I have the tail. You're trying to look at the websites, keep track of the conference calls. Your brain could explode with all the information."

Tellingly, two of the more recent additions to the definition of "information" in the *Oxford English Dictionary* are "information overload" and "information fatigue." Information fatigue is defined as "Apathy, indifference, or mental exhaustion arising from exposure to too much information, esp. (in later use) stress induced by the attempt to assimilate excessive amounts of information from the media, the internet, or at work." As Bowker and Star suggest in their study of classification systems: "The rummage sale of information . . . is overwhelming, and we all agree that finding information is much less of a problem than assessing its quality." Information systems are designed in part, suggest Bowker and Star, not only to store experiences but to connect "experience gained in one time and place with that gained in another, via representations of some sort." This type of context necessarily shifts due to the continual need for encoding and decoding of information to allow for its easy transmission. For Bowker and Star, "information *must* reside in more than one context" for it to be perceived as information at all. To be understood, these different contexts must be "relinked through some sort of judgment." (1999, 7, 290, 291.) It is this linkage that the analysts I worked with performed on a daily basis.

Yet, as Bowker and Star have also argued, "information is only information when there are *multiple* interpretations" and that "it is the tension between contexts that actually creates representation" (1999, 291). In essence, then, there is a permanent tension between the creation of information systems and the increased need for context, between individual and collective interpretation of disease outbreaks and events. Hence it was difficult—if not impossible—for experts to concretely define what they meant by the term "good information," even if good information was seen as being crucial to the daily operations of global public health.

Attempts to Define and Capture Good Information

After a few weeks of tracking all the information traveling into and out of the GDDOC (such as clinical accounts of outbreaks, lab reports on specimen testing, surveillance reports, and emails from team members responding to events), I tried to guess which information would be deemed important or "good" and which would need to be further scrutinized or classified as unimportant or uninteresting. I found that my attempts to play the analyst were usually doomed. In the midst of my own daily confusion about what good information looked like, I began to ask: How do experienced analysts recognize and prioritize information on disease threats?

In global public health, information is sorted using a series of complicated rubrics. Naturally, not all information is viewed as being created equal, so analysts use a variety of qualities and categories to judge information on a scale from "good" to "questionable" to "bad." Information is generally considered "good" when it comes from a known and trusted source, has been scientifically validated (especially in the case of lab results), or has been generated in-house by members of the same national agency. Upon discovery or receipt of information that met this criteria, analysts in the GDDOC generated an internal report on each disease event. The event was then logged into a management system. In essence, such reports were the product of the aggregation and digestion of other prevalidated and already circulating information. Such "information on information" was given a unique ID number, which was used throughout an outbreak, much like a bar coding system for disease agents of the same origin. Events were then shared with other national agencies and all outbreaks were carefully monitored, with information on events updated regularly. In addition to providing a clearing house for "good" information and analysis, the system ensured that no outbreak "went missing."

Any unverified information that filtered into the agency—from any source—would be graded on a scale of credibility, from low to high, using the following formula: credibility of source + validity of information. A high credibility rating would be given to: any information from CDC staff assigned to other countries; information that came from an accepted in-country lab; and any information that had been "verified without line list" (which was basically a catch-all category for all information that came in without any doubt about its authenticity). In essence, if a source was generally seen as competent and trustworthy, or had a history of providing the analysts with valid information, then any information from that source would automatically be granted credibility. On the other hand, information without approved lab confirmation (which usually meant that there was doubt about the authenticity of the information or the trustworthiness and competency of the source) was given a moderate credibility rating. If the source of information had a history of providing valid information most of the time, then the information from that source was also given a moderate credibility rating.

Media and internet sources, and any information that came into the GDDOC without scientific confirmation, were always given a lower credibility rating. Media sources would only be given credibility if the information reported included in-country confirmation of data from a trusted source. Low credibility was also given to any information that lacked context. The quality of information was always partially judged by analysts on the basis of how "logical" it seemed or how "consistent with known events" it was perceived to be compared to the analysts' own experience with the disease agent or the location of the outbreak. Context was needed to help the analysts evaluate the consistency of information from low-credibility sources. Thus, analysts spent most of their time seeking out contextual information to make sense of the hundreds of media and surveillance reports they received on a daily basis. Turning information into "good" information was time-intensive. It required years of experience in order to do quickly and well. Ironically, the so-called solutions to the problem of obtaining good information—increased transparency and the creation of information-sharing networks—simply exacerbated the need for context.

On the Definition of "Context"

While working with epidemiologists and virologists, I often had the distinct impression that they were expressing a desire for something called "perfect information" (Floridi 2010, 98). Perfect information is a term used primarily in game theory to indicate a situation or "game" in which *all* the players have *all* the fundamental information they need to make accurate decisions. Clearly, in the daily practice of epidemiologists and analysts, any individual "player" was almost always playing his or her hand with incomplete information.

As Floridi explains it, in any given situation where there is only imperfect information available, "there is a general need to be able to gain as much as possible of the missing information—either about the players (types, strategies, or payoffs) or the history of the game—by 'retrodicting' (predicting backwards) from the information that one does hold, the information that one misses" (2010, 99). Context is about interpretation as much as it is about "facts on the ground." People expressed a desire for context in order to complete the informational picture about an infectious disease event. In other words, context produced knowledge from incomplete information; it helped to create meaning and thus had a very high value among public health professionals.

Anthropologist and science studies scholar Stefan Helmreich argues that "meaning does not preexist interpretation; rather, the readjustment of context is that which *makes* meaning." Taken from this view, context is not ancillary to the information that it is attached to, but is "woven together" in "a weaving that happens contingently, not deterministically." In an echo of sociologist Harold Garfinkel's thesis that we know what information is only as its usage in a social setting, context in Helmreich's framing "appears as the marker of relevant relations"; it is about what information *does* in a particular setting or environment, not necessarily about what it *is*. (Helmreich 2009, 57, 169, 235.) Context, then, helps us to better see how information is interpreted, how experience and events are woven together to create knowledge about events, and how those using information relate to one another. It is this social view of information that I will take as my departure point for examining context in public health during the 2009 H1N1 pandemic.

The Case of the Missing Context

Near the beginning of the second wave of the pandemic, I attended an international team meeting on H1N1. The meeting started with a slide show of graphs analyzing various data that had recently become available. Most of the data had been circulated in the latest WHO report.

Dr. Marc-Alain Widdowson, the team's leader, announced at the start that they were going to try to start amalgamating information in one location. He told the participants that "We need to try to consolidate all the bits and pieces flying about by email." Almost all those attending nodded. Some smiled and glanced at each other, as if in silent commiseration about the need to reduce the information glut.

The meeting took place as a conference call and lasted about an hour, including a "listen only" period when the director was the only one allowed to speak. Marc-Alain began with an update on the situation in the United States. He seemed to offer up the information as an initial gesture, similar to an opening gift (Malinowski 1922; Mauss 1954). He then gave his personal opinion, based on the data he had just reported: "This will be a bad season, but we knew this already."

Marc-Alain then gave stats on lung infections in ERs, noting that the fall flu season was in "full swing." After he stopped speaking, five people on the conference call gave field reports from regional offices around the world. All were very short and scant in data. There was little to report, and no new activity, since the last call.

While the calls were clearly crucial to the collaborative process of exchanging information and producing meaning, there was an obvious disconnect between what was shared on and off the conference calls, or "on and off the record." It was true that quite a bit of information was readily shared, but not many decisions were made on conference calls. This was a paradox, since the calls were seen as vital to epidemiological sense-making, but were viewed with a mixture of a sense of duty, derision, and apathy by many of the participants. Increasingly, people saw the daily barrage of meetings and conference calls as a waste of their time; they lamented that after months of pandemic response, nothing new was being shared. The real information, the analysts told me—or context—was something one could only get by calling or emailing someone directly and off the record.

In an email later that day, I received the official minutes of the international meeting. The email provided concrete evidence of how people interpreted what they heard, as well as the confusion that might sometimes result from being exposed to different interpretations of the same information. The minutes clearly stated that the upcoming flu season would be a bad one, exactly as the director had opined at the meeting. And yet, something felt missing—a piece of context had dropped out.

Checking my field notes, I found that what Marc-Alain actually said was: "It's going to be a bad season, but we knew this already." How might the elision of the contextual phrase "but we knew this already" alter the meaning of a seemingly objective piece of information about the fall flu season? I suggest that the erasure of Marc-Alain's ancillary "but we knew this already" makes the official statement about the flu season sound more dire than it would have sounded if the reader had been able to access the second half of the director's statement regarding severity. Without the phrase "but we knew this already," we don't know that his statement actually reflects nothing new. There have been no new interpretations, new information, or any developments of real significance. The phrase "but we knew this already" is thus a key piece of contextual information. It indicates that Marc-Alain's thinking about the severity of the upcoming pandemic is more in line with the decreased level of response activity.

In this example, the term "context" is synonymous with "interpretation." What is lost in communication is Marc-Alain's expertise—his personal interpretation of the WHO's data. Without the second part of his statement, or the contextual information, the information about the severity of the upcoming flu season caused a good deal of confusion among those not in attendance at the meeting (such as the other analysts within the GDDOC). The call for more context can thus be read here as an attempt to alleviate some of the uncertainty surrounding the course and severity of the pandemic.

Exchange of Context as Relationship-Building

Uncertainty or doubt about the quality or contents of epidemiological information related to the 2009 H1N1 pandemic were typically dealt with via email. Experts exchanged discrete pieces of information or shared personal opinions and context about already circulating data. In official written communications or reports, all indications of doubt or uncertainty were largely removed. But in more informal communications, experts had more freedom to express doubt or to ask for further clarification about unverified information. These exchanges were most often completed through emails or on smaller conference calls. Not infrequently, however, someone would get frustrated by an inability to explain something adequately in written form and would make an effort to speak directly with a trusted peer—either face-to-face or by calling the person on a private line. When an outbreak of H1N1 in Eastern Europe initially appeared to be unusually severe, the director of the GDDOC phoned a trusted colleague at the WHO for her take on the situation. In this instance, the lab data alone were insufficient; what was required was information on the condition and protocols of the lab that had produced the data and, thus, on its reliability. After speaking with his friend, the director expected that politics had played a role in ramping up the reported threat level, since the country was also in the midst of a hotly contested election.

This exchange of bits of context in an effort to "clear up" uncertain situations, events, or information was part of the analysts' daily routine. The need to fill in gaps in information instigated a great variety of such "context exchanges" between individuals and groups in an effort to understand other information that circulated during the 2009 pandemic. After receiving an email containing lab reports, case counts, or other various epidemiological information, analysts would often contact their colleagues for clarifications or to request the latest updates. In addition to this, the center received many emails, visits, and phone calls for the same purpose and its staff spent a good proportion of their time responding to such enquiries from people working in other divisions or outside of the CDC.

These communications during times of uncertainty were often an integral part of basic relationship-building. The practice of initiating and answering emails and telephone calls helped to strengthen the bonds between individuals who were already familiar with each other and aided in the development of trust between relative strangers. Emails and telephone calls were frequently seen as overtures toward the further development of personal contacts between units or agencies; the analysts would often contact someone for clarification simply to bolster a weak relationship between their team and another division. This type of act was referred to as part of the analyst's job of "staying connected" or "in the loop."

This kind of regular exchange of contextual information had real operational and pragmatic value. Strong ties between individuals and groups meant better access to uncertain information and faster response times. The more robust the personal connections between individual public health professionals, the more quickly future official requests for information would be heeded.

Context, Politics, and "Public Health Diplomacy"

There were instances when it was necessary to provide context in order to smooth over hurt feelings caused by minor disputes over jurisdiction.

The analysts were used to fielding a variety of questions and had learned to be sensitive and diplomatic in their responses. Often it was the analysts who initiated requests for further information, but they also attempted to strengthen their contacts and expand their personal networks by forwarding unasked-for contextual information or analyses to those working in different units or national or international agencies. They often used their tacit knowledge of the intricacies of the global health network to guess who might not have seen or been privy to the agency's vast array of non-public information. Preempting requests for new disease reports or new lab data was an easy way to make those working outside of the agency—especially in other countries—feel less excluded. As a gesture of good faith, this seemingly open and free exchange of new information was, to put it frankly, good for future business.

While working inside the GDDOC, I often felt not completely in the loop myself. Most of what I was given ready access to was surveillance data; I was never privy to the private emails or conversations that occurred in the side communications of the analysts. Whenever people discussed information contained in emails that I hadn't received, I wondered if the omission had been intentional and whether or not the team really trusted me. Questioning the team's trust in me would make me question my own faith in them. My own issues centering on access to information, then, are just one pertinent example of the real emotional effects of feeling in or out of "the loop."

My own experience was not unlike that of the experts I knew. The difference, of course, was that the analysts were highly cognizant of the "chain of command" when communicating with each other, other internal and external divisions, and staff in other countries or national public health institutions. I quickly became interested in mastering this and other protocols and practices that might allow me to gain access to better information and its context myself. To learn more about context, I began to pay more attention to the moments when information flow showed signs of breakdown or friction between various experts. Context exchange was often used during these "incidents" to smooth over any social or political friction.

To Add In or to Not to Add In Context?

While working on the daily H1N1 update, Mike, the team's point person for writing reports on the pandemic, said that he had to be too circumspect in the information that he officially circulated. Because he was the main person who wrote the updates, he felt personally responsible for their content. On this particular occasion, the WHO had released an update on H1N1 in Asia, but Mike was not able to verify everything in the official report—so he was nervous about reporting on it at all.

In response to Mike's query about what to include in the official report, Rohit said, "We're in the business of putting the pieces together. This is the business of risk assessment and projection. We add value by putting things that are speculative into the report."

Later, as I was at my desk trying to compile lists of subject matter experts (SMEs) by disease agent and geographical region (itself a painfully slow context-building task), contention over the wording in the H1N1 update erupted. An SME in influenza from another unit of the CDC, Jane (pseudonym), had contacted Mike to ask him to delete the last paragraph of a report that provided context to the WHO data. The paragraph concerned an outbreak of H1N1 in Europe; it suggested that the localized outbreak might be indicative of the upcoming winter flu season in the temperate zones. Jane argued that the paragraph was "too speculative and confusing." Rohit and Mike had a brief discussion before Mike wrote back to Jane specifying that he would "take her suggestion into consideration," but that the wording in his report had been taken, almost verbatim, from the latest WHO report. Jane sent Mike her own revisions; she wanted to make it clear that it was the WHO speculating, not the GDDOC analysts or SMEs who represented the CDC.

The problem of the interpretation of WHO data was at the core of the dispute over the report's wording. The lab scientists did not want any "speculation" in the report. Public health experts who were not familiar with surveillance methods or analysis, but worked in response or in laboratories, often did not like to circulate anything but verified information, or what they called "hard data." They were not comfortable including guesswork or interpretation—despite the fact that such context was often deemed by others as necessary to the process of turning information into usable knowledge about a disease outbreak. The debate over context here reflects an ever-present tension between a need to wait for "good" information and a need to provide a "best guess" in order to effect response actions. There was thus an endless quest to put available hard data back into context in order to make faster decisions.

Mike and Rohit conferred and decided how best to handle the SME's concerns, and then called their director to make sure that he would "back them up." The director suggested that Mike politely tell Jane that "assessments often contain speculative elements." Mike sent Jane a final response explaining to her that the H1N1 report was not for publication (the report was internal to the agency); that the team always cites their sources; that the last paragraph was speculative but authorized by the WHO; that the paragraph was contextual information that provided valuable perspective on a localized outbreak of particular interest to the international community; and that he had slightly modified the wording of the report to make it obvious that the speculation originated within the WHO itself. The SME was satisfied and the paragraph stayed in the daily report. Mike and Rohit had effectively used context to bolster the agency's own expertise.

Context as Past Experience

One way analysts working in the GDDOC conceptualized the present and tried to anticipate the immediate future was by using their past experiences as a lens to view unfolding events. Every outbreak or piece of information was either overtly or subconsciously linked to something in the past. Sometimes "the past" literally denoted an official historical record of a prior event, but most often it referred to what I call the subjective "experiential rolodex" of respected epidemiologists, scientists, and other experts working in public health. The analysts in the GDDOC often paused in their daily meetings to quietly think to themselves for a moment; they attempted to connect any recollected personal knowledge about similar past events to information about a current outbreak. This type of past-as-context referencing was prevalent during the very beginning of a new outbreak, especially those where the disease agent was still unknown.

In a paradigmatic conversation about a disease outbreak in Country H, Rohit discussed what he remembered from a similar event that took place in Country R in 2001.[3] This was Rohit's attempt to begin to understand— or formulate an opinion about—what was then currently happening in Country H. The past event in Country R provided some insight into how the CDC response team might deal with the event in Country H. However, the comparison—an effort to apply past-referencing context to a new situation—also seemed to constrict the team's choice of response actions.

The fact that the disease agent was known to affect children, was not fatal, and was still of unknown etiology made Rohit hesitant to send assistance to Country H. He was immediately cautious about extending aid to a response project that might last for months (as it had done in Country R), especially if the disease outbreak wasn't an international threat (or likely to spread beyond the borders of Country H). Here the past provided an analytical basis both for thinking about an outbreak in the present and for deciding a course of action to take in the immediate future.

The past as context was a tool generally used by analysts and epidemiologists to "make sense" of current events. Indeed, Rohit explicitly argued that "Building a large database of past cases is important." He explained to me that deciding what should be viewed as a "serious risk" was an art, not a science. It was based almost entirely on contextual information. At a training conference I attended, Rohit explained to the attendees that the job of an analyst in global public health was to understand context. He suggested that "One media report is enough to be concerned, but we look at things contextually. You can't possibly investigate everything—it's a waste of resources. It's like 'crying wolf.' There's no magic number of cases that signals a response—it's context-specific." Because context here is the product of a personal, time-intensive, lived experience with disease outbreaks (and bureaucracies, and budgets, and material limitations), an easy technological fix to the general problem of gathering such contextual information was hard to find.

Context as Value

The more time I spent with the analysts, the less confident I was that there would be any such easy solutions to the problems of real-time information-sharing or collective sense-making. It almost seemed as if the individual users of information were destined to interpret information alone or within small, interpersonal groups. It was unimaginable how technological efforts to design programs that would "capture context"—an idea that had valence almost everywhere I went—would be successful.

People I spoke to were emphatic that "good" information included personal assessments or "gut feelings" regarding so-called hard data. As an epidemiologist working at the WHO suggested during a Berkeley conference on H1N1: "It's not just the hard data, it's the feeling that goes along with it as well. We can communicate the information well, but I'm not sure we can communicate the feeling that goes along with it."

One of her peers at the WHO nodded in agreement, adding: "There's a fair amount of experience in this room, but it's a question of how our gut feelings are translated into information."

A representative from a local California public health agency summed up the problem thus: "It's all personality driven. It all comes back to trust."

The director of the GDDOC, also in attendance at the Berkeley conference, argued that all information-sharing networks required a certain level of trust in order to function at all, stating that "You really have to know who the players are, you really have to know who the organizations are. We were using the term 'social networking' years ago when we were trying to set up networks to get information."

Another top influenza expert added: "Lots of information is not posted anywhere. It's one-to-one, based on trust. I've worked with someone closely in the field and I'll call them up to see what they know or to tell them about what I know."

Some of the public health professionals involved in the 2009 H1N1 pandemic response seemed outwardly dubious about, if not somewhat hostile, to the possibility of sharing such gut-level interpretation more formally or publicly. Context, one epidemiologist at the CDC argued, "is going to be very hard to capture."

There were several reasons that experts were unwilling to share openly what they were willing to share privately. Sharing certain types of sensitive information might get someone in trouble. It was always a personal judgment call, one analyst told me, about "what you share and what you don't." A prominent Hong Kong epidemiologist whom I interviewed likened the sharing of context to office gossip, and declared that "You can sign all kinds of memorandums, but you don't know the guy, and he's not going to tell you anything. It's just like an office. It doesn't happen in a room, but at the water cooler, in the toilet. (*Laughs.*) At the snack bar. During coffee. I think that's a very important point. In these past few years, we've tried very hard to establish good relationships. And trust. So if there's something fishy going on, people are going to tell us." Another epidemiologist echoed this sentiment and equated the sharing of information in global public health to a gift exchange. He suggested that "The response will be quite different for the person coming in with a 'dowry' and those without.

If you call me up and say 'You have anything for me?' the answer is no. But if you come to me with some information, then the response will be very different. Coming in with a 'dowry' will really affect the exchange."

The idea that "good" information or context had an obvious exchange value was echoed many times during conversations with public health professionals regarding their information-sharing practices. Credibility and trust are important attributes of individuals that transfer to the information they share directly. The regular exchange of context as part of "good" information strengthens that same trust and credibility over time. As gifts, these pieces of information and context are "not freely given" and "also not really disinterested" (Mauss 1954, 73). Rather, these informal information-sharing circuits form the basis for the more formal information-sharing systems being set in place by the WHO. The sharing of information informally, especially contextual information, is the foundation for almost all communication. Without these exchanges, communication and sense-making in global public health would be ineffective at best, and grind to a halt at worst.

The Informational Hierarchy of Resort

The GDDOC analysts had separate areas of expertise: virology, bacteriology, parasitology, zoonotic disease. If they didn't know about a disease agent from direct personal experience or knowledge, then they researched it. When I asked each of them to explain how they collected information on outbreaks or disease agents, they mentioned that they usually brought their own personal networks to bear on their jobs as analysts. These contacts were from their past—a mixture of work relationships or friendships cemented during time in school, while working at previous jobs, or in the course of completing the CDC's prestigious two-year fellowship in the Epidemiological Intelligence Service program. The analysts relied heavily upon these networks for "good" information and for clarification of any uncertain information. The people concerned were typically not on the SME contact list that the team usually used for vetting events within the CDC; it was much faster to get information from informal sources whom the analysts already knew to be reliable. Personal contacts were always the first resort when further information or context were needed.

If the analysts could not obtain "good" information from friends and personal contacts, then they expanded their search accordingly. Avoiding what was generally referred to as "official sources" or formal contacts, analysts would seek out colleagues in the GDDOC—or the people whom they knew well—and ask them for an introduction to their own personal contacts in the subject area required. Relying upon a close colleague's contacts, however, added a layer of difficulty to the task of gathering information. As an example, someone who was a personal contact for Rohit would still be a stranger to Kira, and Rohit's contact might be hesitant to divulge any "unofficial" information to her. Yet team members still conceptualized using contacts of contacts as being far easier than extracting information from more official, formalized sources.

What the analysts did, in essence, was to tap into the relationships already set up by their own. Ergo, trust Rohit had built with his sources was extended—by proxy of Kira's relationship to Rohit—to Kira herself. The flexible expansion of personal networks here had the effect of making Rohit's contacts feel more comfortable telling Kira—a relative stranger— something "off the record." From what I observed inside the GDDOC, the practice of relying upon what I will label here as "second-order contacts" was an immense help both in procuring contextual information and in forging new relationships and strengthening existing information-sharing networks.

The last resort for gathering information is the official network. One of the younger analysts on the team, Kira, admitted that she would only contact someone from the official SME list if she could not find the information anywhere else. The official level, she explained, was where she found the most "obstacles" to getting what she needed. Indeed, all the analysts told me that people could be tricky at this level of interaction, where the amount of accrued personal trust was low because the individuals had little or no prior experience working with one another. Social friction, or what members of the analyst team frequently referred to as "dealing with personalities," was viewed as being heightened by formal protocols of information-sharing inside larger global health networks. As a result, people were stingy with their information—especially if it had not yet been "verified." Essentially, what was described to me is—and here I borrow shamelessly from Arthur Kleinman's use (1980) of Lola Romanucci-Ross's original concept (1977)—a "hierarchy of resort" for information gathering.

The epidemiologists I worked with had a hierarchy of preferred sources for obtaining information.

Ancillary to the problem of sourcing and access to information was the problem of "on the record" or public exchanges versus "off the record" or back-channel sharing of context and information. Not only did epidemiologists working as analysts in global public health have to spend an inordinate amount of time sourcing, confirming, and assessing information, they also had to repackage information (adding in analysis and context) in order to circulate it back into the information-sharing network or "loop." This concept of the "information loop" was raised many times in my conversations with experts in regard to gaining access to "good" information. It could be difficult, if not impossible, to get access to information shared "off the record."

Most of the analysts were vigilant about having all email conversations take place "online"—meaning that the other analysts on the team, as well as contacts in other units or within separate public health or governmental agencies, were "kept in the loop" through the diligent use of email "cc's" and the use of a group mailbox. This mailbox would receive an email message and autoforward it to a list of names set by the GDDOC staff. Because it was seen as vital that all analysts and agency staff work on the basis of the same information, the analysts made strong attempts to forward any "offline" (informal, unofficial, or even in-person) replies to group emails. However, if things were especially busy or an analyst became distracted by another task, he could forget to do this altogether and then the other analysts might complain that they were "out of the loop."

Throughout the 2009 H1N1 pandemic, public health practitioners viewed the problems of "being in the loop" and of what I refer to here as the informational hierarchy of resort as dual obstacles to effective communication and the ability to do their jobs. On the one hand, everyone spoke about "good" information as though its definition were part of a collective tacit knowledge. In reality, however, different people working in different agencies and in different units all had access to different information and slightly different definitions of "good" information—from both a qualitative and quantitative standpoint. In part, this is due to the fact that different public health agencies have different operational environments and cultures. These cultural differences, in turn, make any easy technological solution to the problem of obtaining "good" information next to impossible. What might be needed instead is a better working definition of good information and the development of what I call Good Information Technology.

The Anthropology of Good Information

As someone argued to me, echoing a statement that I heard from nearly everyone I met working on the 2009 H1N1 response: "The data were crap. I mean, that's it. Because it's very, very difficult to gather the information that you need." This powerful and provocative statement—that the information being circulated transparently and rapidly through the official public health networks is not good enough—was often coupled with the suggestion that there is "too much" information being produced in the first place. I soon came to believe that what was at stake in these dirges about a lack of "good" information was the very definition of information in public health.

The problem of defining good information, the data deluge, and examples of the role of context above should be read together as an ethnography of the daily practice of turning information into actionable knowledge within epidemiology. They also highlight the various problems of attempts to gather, analyze, and report good information on H1N1 throughout the 2009 pandemic. But perhaps most importantly, these examples are indicative of the messy and complex process of making sense out of a daily barrage of information. Without context, information is essentially useless to those tasked with making decisions about public health response. Understanding what these experts mean when they talk about the need for more context, then, is key not only to examining and analyzing public health networks themselves or the way they function, but is crucial to developing methods to foster stronger communication and trust among various partners in global public health. The stakes are high; without actionable knowledge, experts must make "good enough" decisions. "Bad" information can be disastrous. In the case of rapidly spreading infectious diseases, the difference between an outbreak and a deadly pandemic may rest upon experts (such as the analysts discussed above) having access to the good information they need to make the best possible response decisions.

To deal with the increasing volume of data and information, health organizations utilize a set of criteria for determining "good" information and have developed a protocol for information-sharing. Yet the epidemiologists who work within large public health institutions and agencies still have to individually make sense of each unique situation by using that set of criteria as a guideline. In order for certain response decisions and actions to take place, epidemiologists must rely upon each other's analyses and personal judgments. The use of context captured from my fieldwork and described above suggests to me that information in global public health moves through the following informational "life stages":

1. *Information gathering*, or aggregating data from unofficial, surveillance, or informal sources
2. *The search for context*, or understanding and analyzing all previously aggregated information in light of personal opinions, unvalidated information, or contextual details of disease outbreaks
3. *Production, (re)circulation, and utilization of "good" information* to affect official response actions or recommendations for local actions

While information on an outbreak might look exactly the same, the contextual information produced by people who interpret that information is necessarily different. In other words, *different conclusions will be based on the same information* (see chapter 3 on quarantine for just one pertinent example). This difference is qualitative and due to the common daily practice of producing contextual information that is itself based on the unique lived experiences of individuals working in public health. It is this type of *past, lived experience as context* that global public health information systems have trouble sharing through any formal channels. The multitude of teleconferences, meetings, emails, and personal telephone calls that I observed throughout my fieldwork are attempts to gather such experiences as context—all in a concerted, if misplaced, effort to qualify and quantify what it was difficult for many individuals to describe, let alone to capture in an email or standardized form.

While some studies have paid attention to how various experts, such as the analysts discussed here, gather and consume information, little attention has been paid to the human/technology interface that produces such information in the first place. One solution might be to take the production and use of so-called good information and the development of information technologies to capture these more seriously from an anthropological viewpoint. In other words, we need to do more work in the anthropology of good information. Back in the early 1990s, we started attending to what Arturo Escobar called the nascent "anthropology of cyberculture" (1994) and others termed "cyborg anthropology" (American Anthropological Association 1993). The anthropology of information is nothing new per se, but maybe we need to examine the ways in which an anthropology of "good" information might be different and why.

Of course, scholars have already begun doing this: Dominic Boyer's work on "the information practices" of journalism and anthropology—all of us "sharing a 'life informatic'" (2005, xi); Gabriella Coleman's work on hackers and hacking culture (2012); Chris Kelty's body of work in the "post-internet" era (Kelty 2008), looking at "the circulation and authorization of knowledge of all kinds" (Fischer et. al., 2008, 560); ethnographies and scholarly examinations of digital social media (Boellstorff 2008, Miller 2011, Turkle 2011). What I hope to invigorate here is a continuation of what Brenda Laurel and Joy Mountford originally called "interface anthropology" (1990): ethnographic accounts of how humans develop and use information technology, or what that technology allows users *to do* and what it *does to them*.

We also need to collectively rethink what we mean by the term "information." As social scientists, we haven't gone much further than Harold Garfinkel's exploration of the concept ([1952] 2008); his premise that we can only know what the thing "information" is by attending to its usages in social settings is a good place to start. Information is a social fact, a social product, a social building block. It *is* the network. Epidemiologists, in essence, want new technologies that can produce better information—what I will call a collective desire for the development of Good Information Technology. What if we took the idea of Good Information Technology seriously? Could we have an anthropology of good information—or contextualized information—to go along with it?

The resultant "anthropology of good information" would pay particular attention to points where the human and the technological become enmeshed with each other in the process of sense-making. As Bowker and Star have argued, there is "a permanent tension between universal standardization" of information-sharing systems and "the local circumstances of those using them" (1999, 139). Efforts at further standardization of information technology in global public health are only doomed to worsen the problem if they fail to take the problem of context more seriously; and context is best understood at the level of the social and the cultural.

Heretical Contexts

In the next and final chapter, I explore the narratives of a small collection of scientists who identify as infectious disease experts, but realize that their personal opinions regarding the best future direction of microbiological research go against the current reigning research paradigm. In essence, they are outsider/insiders who argue that viruses are not necessarily the enemies of the human race that they are often made out to be. In defining their life's work, these men tell a different tale about man and microbes—one that has less to do with opposition and war metaphors and more to do with cohabitation and understanding. Read against their more "orthodox" brethren, these "heretics" and their stories highlight not only how intimately scientists relate to their objects of study, but help us to see how the narrative of the 2009 H1N1 pandemic is continuously negotiated among individuals with differing opinions, status as experts, past experiences, and beliefs about the threat posed by the influenza virus. In sum, the next chapter explores how scientists deploy their own personal "contexts" to interpret events and argue for certain courses of action over others.

7

THE HERETICS OF MICROBIOLOGY

Charisma, Expertise, Disbelief, and the Production of Knowledge

If you're a chicken, the H5N1 virus is a very bad virus.

DR. PETER PALESE, virologist

Gene Segment M. Biological Function: *The matrix protein (M) segment actually encodes for two separate proteins (M1 and M2) and may be involved in determining influenza's host tropism (the process that determines which cells a virus is capable of infecting). The evolution of the M segment is thought to reflect host-specific adaptation; evolutionary virologists compare the genetic makeup of M segments in strains infecting humans and birds in an effort to understand how Influenza A viruses adapt to their hosts. The M protein is also a target of recent efforts at developing a universal vaccine for influenza.* Pathographic function: *This segment of the pathography might easily have been its beginning. The personal and individual narratives of experts examined below not only reflect the underlying scientific paradigm that drives influenza surveillance and research programs, but also reveals how viral expertise is continuously crafted and negotiated within the global network. Although the interpretation of data on influenza changes depending on whom you ask, the need for basic research on the virus remains unquestioned. Ultimately, this chapter explores how our collective understanding of influenza is based upon a productive juxtaposition of scientific knowledge about the virus and differing expert opinions about what facts about flu actually mean.*

In the Greek myth of Cassandra, the god of prophecy—Apollo—adorns his beloved with the gift of foresight and then, after she has spurned him, curses her to be forever ignored and mistrusted. Messages to her people, the Trojans, about what will befall them if they continue their various courses of action go unheeded; yet Cassandra never stops speaking her truth, never ceases in her attempts to compel the Trojans to heed her warnings. Only after the Trojans fall to the Greeks does she finally retreat into the temple of Athena—seeking protection from the goddess of wisdom and reason, though even reason cannot save her from her fate. Cassandra's prescience, and her inability to communicate her vision of the future, is a ripe metaphor for at the situation of global public health experts in the twenty-first century.

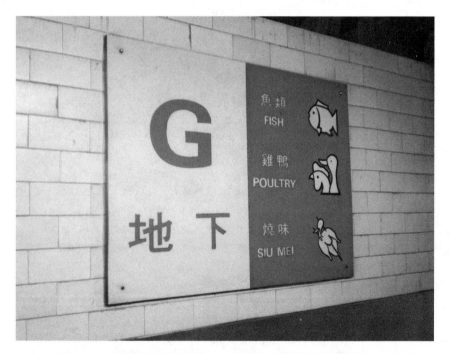

Figure 13. A sign from the now-closed wet market in Central District, Hong Kong. Photo taken in 2008.

The phrase "not if, but when"—often used in preparedness talks to describe the possibility of another global scourge as dire as the medieval plagues—has been uttered so many times by so many different biosecurity and health experts that it has become devoid of almost all meaning. "Not if, but when" has become the standard cry in response to an uncertain future—as readily deployed in the twenty-first century as Cassandra's prophecies to the Trojans. But what to make of this hollowed-out phrase? And why do so many continue to deploy it as a rationale for increased funding for global disease surveillance and response?

In this chapter, I examine the two major ways in which experts working on influenza in global public health think of themselves in relationship to their peers and to the microbes they have spent the greater part of their lives studying. The first is to see oneself as an insider-outsider who speaks against the reigning scientific paradigm. I refer to these scientists as the "heretics" of microbiology because they see themselves as speaking against common conceptions of disease and human health. The second is to see oneself as part of a group of public health experts that continuously warn against the threat of future pandemics but whose words and recommendations go unheeded, either by "laymen" or by inexpert government officials. These are the "orthodox." In either formulation, the experts do not have "neutral" relationships to influenza or to other infectious disease agents. To hearken back to chapter 1 of this book, virologists and epidemiologists are in intimate relationships with the microbes that they study, as well as in complicated relationships with each other and with the public.

Global public health is a distinct society; it has its own rules, norms, habitus, customs, beliefs, and ways of thinking about disease. In the end, I came to understand the 2009 pandemic as a type of interactive drama writ large (Goffman 1959, Hilgartner 2000). Scientific experts perform not only for the public or for government officials, but for each other.

But if the pandemic was a partial performance, then what I observed might best be considered as a type of epidemiological "front"—or, as Goffman suggests, a "collective representation" that is "a fact in its own right." The scientists and epidemiologists I worked with were indeed hyperaware of the established roles that they were expected to perform (in regard to their colleagues, their superiors, and to the public). Sometimes they went against a standard performance or deviated from their prescribed roles. Indeed, it is the heretic's role as part of a collective performance that allows him to cause so much "trouble" for the team in the first place. (Goffman 1959, 27, 83.)

This is why I linger with the heretics. It is not just that I find their personal charisma compelling enough to believe in their opinions over those of their more orthodox brethren. It is because as exceptions they provide me with an interesting way to interrogate what is accepted as "common knowledge" in global public health. The heretics' resistance to the collective wisdom that influenza is always already a serious threat, and that microbes should be considered as the enemy, is indicative of an emergent counterparadigmatic narrative. Yet it also undergirds the master narrative of influenza as an important object for scientific research and knowledge production. The heretics and the orthodox might disagree on the meaning of influenza research, but they agree on the importance of the research itself. Thus, as we will see below, the exception does indeed sometimes prove the rule.

Into a Heretic's Den

Among the leading heretics regarding the imminence and seriousness of the avian influenza pandemic threat is none other than the biologist in whose lab I received my tuition in sequencing procedures, Professor Frederick C. Leung. Through our email conversations before I arrived in Hong Kong, I already knew that he held a strong, albeit controversial, conviction that some scientists, epidemiologists, and public health officials had taken the wrong tack in regard to influenza, the vaccination of animal populations and humans, and the culling of animals who were found to have the highly pathogenic form of the "dangerous" H5N1 virus. He felt that officials—and some scientists—were overreacting, that they didn't understand the virus. In short, Fred Leung did not think that avian influenza was the threat it was made out to be.

Fred Leung was one of the first people in Hong Kong to respond to my request for a personal interview. Most everyone else seemed to be assiduously trying to avoid talking to me. An outsider to the realm of public health, despite my time working inside the CDC, I had difficulty in accessing the inner circle of infectious disease experts in Hong Kong. This was so much the case that I became habituated to emailing and telephoning virologists and government public health officials with delayed or no response. I knew from the beginning, then, that Fred might be different from his peers.

Fred Leung's office, like those of so many professors, was stacked ceiling to floor with manila folders, books, articles, and printout sheets of sequencing data. There were a dehumidifier and a fan running in the corner, and pictures of his family adorning one wall. His office was located just down the hall from his lab on the fifth floor of the Kadoorie Biological Sciences Building. A quote about being a great teacher hung on the wall above his computer. Prof. Leung had graying hair and wire-rimmed glasses yet was spry in his movements. When he met me, he jumped up from his chair to give me a warm, firm handshake. In our first interview, he laughed often, and often at himself. I immediately found this disarming. It was as if he knew that he had no one else to blame for whatever troubles he might have, and yet was happy with his lot.

Over the span of a few months, we covered so many topics that it would be impossible for me to go into them in detail here, or even to summarize. Our conversations were disjointed—much as if we were two viruses swapping information haphazardly in the same host. It was a necessary function to find out what each of us knew and what each of us might discover from the other. Obviously, Fred had far more knowledge about the viruses themselves; he has been living in the medium of infectious zoonotic viruses so long that he talked for hours without getting anywhere in particular. During our first encounter, Fred threw his hands up in the air and said, "You want stories? I've got plenty of stories."

Taped on the back of his door was a long, narrow phylogeny chart of a segment of H5N1, where he had highlighted various segments that had been found in samples taken from humans infected with the virus. He shook his head as he explained the various parts to me and said: "What this says to me is that it's totally random." What he meant was that no particular genetic part of the RNA could be considered *the* gene segment responsible for bird-to-human transmission. In other words, Fred did not believe in the focus on sequencing particular gene segments considered by other experts as key to the virus's replication and transmission (in essence, the gene segments that coded for the hemagglutinin (H) and neuraminidase (N) proteins). Because of his controversial viewpoints, Fred's career had not blossomed as much as those of his counterparts and colleagues in Hong Kong.

On our very first day, Fred said, "You know about the influenza mafia, right?"

I didn't know what he meant or how to answer him, so I simply shook my head.

"The WHO, the CDC, they are like the mafia. There are unwritten codes of conduct. They control funding or whether or not something gets published. Of course, I have no proof of this. But I know. Now tell me, if that isn't the mafia, then what is?" He paused, then laughed.

In essence, Fred believes that influenza surveillance is a big machine, a moneymaker for public health agencies and labs, and is filled with scientists seeking to gain both credibility and funding for their work. It is, in Fred's estimation, an unstoppable research paradigm. To do anything differently would be to admit that they—the influenza experts—were wrong, and Fred often assured me that neither the WHO nor the CDC would do that anytime soon. They have bought into a system, Fred argues, and that system supports them. For better or for worse, the "influenza mafia" is here to stay. Fred, with a substantially lower level of funding and scant access to tissue samples collected by those working either within or closely with government health agencies, works on the fringe of this "mafia-controlled" scientific territory.

As I pondered Fred's marginal role in the global influenza network and his outspokenness about the direction of flu research, I found myself reverting to Erving Goffman's conceptualization of those who play the social role of the outsider. Goffman argues that "Renegades often take a moral stand, saying that it is better to be true to the ideals of the role than to the performers who falsely present themselves in it." In Fred Leung's case, his motivation for continuing to collect and sequence influenza viruses was to expose what he saw as the partially self-interested science of influenza surveillance and research. By the end of my fieldwork, I came to view Fred, and those of a similar mindset, as exemplars of Goffman's "defrocked priests," those who "tell us what goes on in the monastery." (Goffman 1959, 165, 164.) Heretical "confessions" are of particular interest in relation to the creation and operation of more orthodox ways of thinking about influenza within networks of viral expertise. Using Goffman, Stephen Hilgartner reminds us that the scientific credibility of experts is "produced in social action." Virologists and epidemiologists, then, "use a variety of dramatic techniques to create—or better, to *enact*—the basis of their authority as experts." Protagonists—or orthodox experts like Robert Webster or Keiji Fukuda—give narrative structure to pandemic events and respond to or "preempt" opposing stories, like those of Fred Leung. (Hilgartner 2000, 7, 6.) Thus, stage management during events such as the 2009 H1N1 pandemic—à la Goffman—is part and parcel of expert authority. Performers actively reveal or conceal information in order to control the pandemic narrative—indeed, the control of epidemiological information is tightly related to the performance of scientific expertise. As Hilgartner argues, "struggles to control access to information are an integral part of struggles over the creation of knowledge" (2000, 20). Credibility here is networked; expertise emerges from the relationships between orthodoxy and heterodoxy.

For science studies scholars Collins and Evans, expertise is not simply "relational," but "real," even if attaining expertise is ultimately a "social process." Expertise is not simply the product of experts' relationships with each other; there is, Collins and Evans suggest, something *substantive* about it. It is not wholly socially constructed. Like Collins and Evans, I am interested, ultimately, in how experience, or local and personal context, can affect expertise. They argue that if the "speed of politics exceeds the speed of scientific consensus formation," then we—as a society—need to become more comfortable with using incomplete or "fallible" science to act. (Collins and Evans 2007, 2, 3, 8.) In other words, if we are forced to rely on best guesses during an influenza pandemic, we had better know who the best experts are to make those guesses for us. Those best guesses will be, typically, based on some admixture of experience (context) *and* expertise. But what, then, might we learn from the heretics in influenza science that might help us better understand how we come to construct, rely upon, and utilize scientific knowledge to make decisions? The next section reflects upon what counts as "experience" in the first place and how we might include something like *heretical expertise* as a category of expertise in and of itself.

Charisma, Belief, and the Production of Heretical and Orthodox Expertise

Scholars who study science have problematized any easy division between the realms of scientific knowledge—or "facts"—and belief. Maintaining a strict distinction between "doxa" (opinion) and "episteme" (knowledge) (Callon, Lascoumes, and Barthe 2009, 99) is particularly problematic in relationship to events or phenomena that are uncertain—such as viruses or global pandemics. To be scientific, it is generally agreed upon, a researcher must break with opinion. However, as science studies scholars Callon, Lascoumes, and Barthe have argued, this division between opinion and knowledge—which is tricky to sustain at the best of times—is especially blurry in relationship to an event like the 2009 H1N1 pandemic wherein certainty or actionable information is scant. They suggest instead that "Science and passion, knowledge and identities are inseparable and co-evolving" (2009, 106). Scientists are, of course, mortal human beings—ones who rely upon both knowledge and opinion to formulate expert decisions about the future risk of a deadly influenza pandemic. But the real difference between the orthodox and the heretics of influenza science lies not in their opinions about the value of influenza research or its products per se, but in the construction of different types of knowledge.

In what follows, I will show that within the realm of global influenza networks, both heretics and orthodox operate on the basis of the same doxa: they both hold similar and deeply ingrained beliefs and values that inform their actions as influenza researchers and epidemiologists. As Pierre Bourdieu argues:

> ... the censorship exercised by orthodoxy—and denounced by heterodoxy—conceals a more radical censorship which is also harder to detect because it is constitutive of the very functioning of the field, and because it bears on the totality of what is admitted by the mere fact of belonging to the field, and on the totality of what is set beyond discussion by the mere fact that the agents accept the issues at stake in argument, i.e., the consensus on the objects of dissensus, the common interests underlying conflicts of interest, all the undiscussed and unthought areas tacitly kept outside the *limits* of the struggle. (2004, 41)

Or, to state things in different terms, what is beyond argument in global public health and networks of viral expertise is the value of studying influenza viruses in the first place. The field of influenza science itself is never questioned. The quality of expertise about the influenza virus may be debated, but the action of studying influenza viruses is not.

In this section, I place the narratives of the heterodoxy in conversation with those of the orthodoxy to highlight not only how the two overlapping groups might differ in their interpretation of the meaning of influenza research, but how personal charisma plays an integral role in the creation of expertise writ large. The personal charisma of the heretics and the charismatic allure of the orthodox are tools deftly deployed in order to gain support for distinct visions of the future of influenza science—or molecular biology—itself. The stories told here interweave the past, future, and lived present during the 2009 H1N1 pandemic and highlight how expertise is continuously constructed. Events within these tales—and their meanings—are constantly being negotiated and are constantly in flux. As much as interpretations of the science may differ, however, the underlying scientific research paradigm is never problematized. In the end, it is the very friction between these heretical and orthodoxical accounts that reifies influenza as a legitimate scientific object of study.

Heretical Tales: Exaggerated Risk, Fear-Mongering, and the Need for Basic Science

Fred Leung began his career as an endocrinologist. After receiving his Ph.D. from Berkeley in 1978, he spent the next two decades working and researching within the fields of biochemistry and animal science. Upon returning to his native Hong Kong, he took up a post at the University of Hong Kong, first in zoology, then as dean of sciences, and—in his most recent and current position—as a full professor of biological sciences. He is the supervisor of HKU's Evolutionary and Molecular Biology Group, and his research centers on animal and human viruses, viral evolution, chicken genome molecular epidemiology, and phylogenetic characterization and analysis of agriculturally important animal viruses such as avian influenza and the virus that causes foot and mouth disease. Throughout his career, Leung has contributed over two hundred gene sequences to Genbank (the NIH-run genetic sequence database) and published over a hundred peer-reviewed journal articles.

When I met Fred Leung in the spring of 2010, his lab at HKU was busy sequencing different viruses from farms around Hong Kong, the New Territories, and southern China. In addition, the lab was working on the development of vaccines for agriculturally important viruses (such as foot and mouth disease). Over the years, Fred had developed an intensive relationship with a small network of local duck, chicken, and pig farmers who would regularly call him whenever outbreaks occurred and consistently relied upon his expertise and confidentiality. In return, Fred was fiercely loyal to them and spoke proudly about the level of trust that had grown up between the lab and the farmers. Fred often came into friendly conflict with government officials when they asked him to disclose the locations of farms from which his samples were collected.

Fred repeatedly warned me, when I made arrangements to observe his lab and to interview him, that he was not orthodox in his beliefs about the threat of H5N1. He worried about my research and constantly gave me suggestions about whom else to interview on the subject. In essence, he wanted me to have both sides of the story, so that I could judge for myself.

The following is a conversation I had with Fred in his office during early March 2010. I had recently begun fieldwork in Hong Kong. This particular exchange was recorded, and centered on the history of influenza research in the city. The narrative that Fred constructs below interlaces the past with the future in the present moment to explain his belief that the threat of both H5N1 and H1N1 had—and have—been exaggerated. He relied upon his own expertise to undergird his arguments. He also peppered our conversation with outbursts of laughter and self-mocking. In fact, he was very charming. We began our talk with a history lesson as backdrop to our conversation about the 2009 pandemic:

> *Fred Leung:* When SARS first broke out in Hong Kong, they were looking for H5 for two weeks. Every morning they [public health authorities in the city] had conference calls with the WHO, asking: "Any positive samples?" No. After about a week and a half, they knew they were on the wrong track. But the WHO was ready to ring that bell. They were just about to hit the pandemic bell and say, "See? We told you so!"
>
> *TM:* But every year seasonal flu kills so many people.
>
> *FL:* Exactly. But most of those people die from secondary infections. Not the flu. We spend billions of dollars [on surveillance and vaccine research], and we're just not getting anywhere. Not going anywhere! The whole thing

about viruses, we are misguided, in my own opinion. Politicians buy into the system, drug companies buy into it, they make money, and nobody says anything, they just ride the wave. Because it thrives on human fears and it is a perfect unknown scenario. So they can never hang you on it. But H5 is different. Because they went one step further—predicting. That's the problem, you see?

Fred's suggestion that an avian influenza pandemic cannot be predicted is reminiscent of evolutionary virologists' concerns in chapter 1 that genealogical information about a particular circulating virus should not be used to predict that virus's development in the future. It is important to point out here that the heretical and orthodox views on science's ability to foresee emerging viruses are very similar.[1]

Heretic experts like Fred do not believe that H5N1 or other strains of avian influenza, like H7N9 and their descendants, are a "true" pandemic-level threat; while orthodox experts, such as Stephen Morse and Robert Webster, very much do think so. As the "father" of influenza research as we know it, Webster believes that avian influenzas are "not so benign" (1993, 41).[2] Their mutability—their ability to both genetically drift over time or suddenly shift—concerns him. Webster, and those many experts who subscribe to this version of the "influenza narrative," argue that avian influenzas like H5N1 are capable of mutating into deadlier forms. Although heretics such as Fred recognize influenza's unique capability to evolve, they do not buy into the narrative that Influenza A viruses will necessarily or inevitably cause another 1918-like pandemic. As Fred explained it:

Look, I know the [H5] virus is very bad. If it's a virulent strain, 24-hours. Less than 24 hours. You look at the bird, and the bird starts rolling its eyes, you really can see if that virus is a high-path virus. But I have asked Guan Yi[3] all these years about samples that he collected from healthy or not-sick birds. . . . How are you going to convince me that this is high-path? He said, "No! We put it in the chicken eggs and the chicken embryo died!" But no one can explain to me why that happened, but the bird itself didn't get sick. And we sequenced that virus and it didn't have the basic amino acid for high-path. And I even asked Bob Webster, and he couldn't answer this.

Guan Yi refuses to talk to me now. His postdocs scream at my students. They ask us: "Why are you saying they don't need to kill the chickens?"

We used to have 500 chicken farms and 500 pig farms in the area. Right now, March 9, 2010, there are 29 chicken farms and 43 pig farms. Sad case, in my opinion. The social impact is that everybody pays a higher price for fresh meat.

They keep talking about how bad [viral] reassortment is. Yes, there is danger, but we don't know the exact risk or hazard. And the fear, in my opinion, is exaggerated. You know, those so-called signature sequences misled so many people. Everybody was doing selective listening.

The "signature sequences" referenced above are the genetic sequences for the two protein molecules H (hemagglutinin) and N (neuraminidase), particularly those of the infamous 1918 H1N1 influenza strain. Representing the orthodox view, Robert Webster argues that the H and N proteins are of "special importance" (1993, 37). The H and N proteins are key to the influenza virus's ability to get into and out of a host cell. In Webster's own influential research on influenza A virus strains, he argues that minor changes—referred to as "point changes"—in the H protein alone make the difference between a "mild" virus and a deadly one (1993, 42). As a result, the genetic sequences of H and N proteins have become central to the orthodox influenza surveillance and research paradigm.

Yet Fred Leung is not alone in his assessment that influenza experts like Webster are "misled" by similarities in H and N proteins. Evolutionary biologist Paul W. Ewald is another heretic scientific expert who believes it is a logical mistake to assume that the H and N proteins are what make any particular influenza viral strain dangerous. Ewald suggests that while the H and N proteins are the two proteins that are most visible to the human immune system, there is no reason to believe that they are responsible for any particular strain's pathogenicity or severity. Ewald argues that scientists often confuse "sources of variation—the mutation and recombination of genes—with the process of evolution by natural selection," and worries that spending too much time looking for a repeat of the 1918 pandemic strain is a waste of epidemiological resources. (Ewald 2000, 22–23, 25.) To borrow Charles Rosenberg's phrasing, what Leung and Ewald are suggesting is that the public health orthodoxy has become too ready to see what it has already been prepared to look for and to fear (see chapter 4). Past pandemics such as that of 1918 are used within heretical narratives of expertise to suggest that the more orthodox use of the same history is flawed. The history is used to create, in essence, a heretical expertise to oppose the orthodoxy's version of influenza's threat.

In addition to being cautious about "signature sequences," Fred Leung is also producing and articulating a different type of knowledge here. Intertwined with his interpretation of gene segments is an embedded cultural knowledge about the effects of culling farm animals like chickens and pigs on the population of Hong Kong, the New Territories, and Guangdong Province. Leung discusses the social and economic impact of frequent culling practices on the communities in which he works and lives. This is a different mode of concern for human well-being—and of knowledge production—from those of Guan Yi, Robert Webster, and others who share concerns dissimilar to Leung's related to an assumed greater future pathogenicity of bird flu in humans. For Guan Yi and Webster, the loss of chickens and pigs in China is a small price to pay for safety, even if that measure of safety is uncertain in terms of its overall effectiveness in preventing a deadly pandemic. For Fred, however, these practices have a very high cost. Fred self-consciously brings a scientific *and* a social knowledge to his work and thereby crafts a different type of heretical expertise.

Despite Leung's incorporation of a daily, lived, social experience into his research, scientific knowledge about the influenza virus remains the bulwark of both categories of expertise. Heretics no less than orthodox rely upon the soundness of their science to make claims about influenza. The practice of genetic sequencing itself is not seen as the problem within these dueling narratives. Rather, it is the *interpretation* of genetic data that is at stake in both sets of narratives. In the following conversation, Fred Leung explained the importance of continued sequencing in the global quest to better understand the influenza virus:

> FL: In 1997, when I first returned [from the United States], I had the first sequencing machine at HKU, and I offered to sequence H5N1. They sent it instead to the US CDC. After we had the big outbreak [of H5N1], I went to visit Bob Webster. Of course he is a prominent scientist, and I am just a (*uses hand to indicate a lower level*). But back in 1999, everybody was just doing H and N sequencing. That's it. I told Bob that I thought we needed to do full genome sequencing in order to really understand this virus. And then he started collaborating with other people and

began doing full genome sequencing and came up with the concept of recombinations.

TM: Do you think sticking to your guns about H5N1 has hurt your
        career?

FL: Oh, definitely. But I'm a very good teacher. At this university,
        I've been given the teaching award. So what is your priority in
        life—what is important? I spend time with my family. And every
        hour you spend with them is one less hour to do other things. Of
        course, quantitatively, it has had an impact on my research.

    And of course when I said that you don't need to kill the
chickens, and the former health minister [Margaret Chan] gave
the order to kill all the chickens and now she's the head of the
WHO. . . . And you think that that doesn't impact me, in terms of
research? Hah! Of course it does. Why does my proposal always
get rejected? No funding. Now, of course I have no proof. And
I accept that this is the way it is. However, the beautiful thing is,
I still can say what I believe in, irrespective. And that is enough.
That is enough. And what is truth, anyway? Truth gets milled in.
What is important is one's own priority, one's own principle.

    Has the risk of a deadly pandemic gone away? No. It's the
same risk, in my opinion. But it's not a bird problem, it's not a
pig problem, it's not a bat problem, it's not an animal problem.
It's just politics. It's a problem with the signal. You see, it's about
detectable level. When your sensitivity is high, then the numbers
get magnified. Fifty years ago, viruses crossing over from animals
to humans never amounted to anything. This is why we have
all these "new" viruses—because our sequencing technology is *so*
powerful. We can sequence a whole genome in one week. That's
the problem. You detect the signal you are looking for.

TM: So then what does all the sequencing data mean? Why keep se-
        quencing flu viruses?

FL: I can tell you what it means, because I'm a true believer in knowl-
        edge. (*Long pause.*) It's a goldmine. No, it's not a goldmine. That's
        not the right metaphor. (*Short pause.*) It's like oil in the ground.
        I'm a true believer in sequencing viruses. It's all black oil.

Fred Leung's assertion that scientific research on influenza viruses should
continue is not at odds with more orthodox views on the need for continual viral surveillance and genetic sequencing. As he states, he is a "true
believer" in the science of sequencing. The data are like a deep reservoir of

knowledge that can be mined or tapped into by subsequent generations of scientists. What the genetic information cannot tell virologists now might tell them something in the future. This continual delay of knowledge does nothing to preclude the slow accrual of expertise about the virus in the present; in fact, it intensifies it. Sequencing in influenza labs contributes to a pool of data that can be interpreted differentially to produce different types of knowledge about flu. For scientists like Fred Leung, this "oil" might lead to the proof the heretics need to undergird their argument that highly pathogenic influenza viruses naturally burn themselves out, that they pose no greater risk to humanity than "normal" influenza viruses. For scientists like Robert Webster, however, the interpretation of the same set of data might lend them proof that influenza viruses like H5N1 are as dangerous as the orthodoxy claims that they are.

To go back to Bourdieu, then, the underlying doxa is the same. Viruses should be randomly sampled, sequenced, and studied. The episteme that is produced from this genetic information, however, is qualitatively different. Influenza viruses are dangerous or they are not; we need avian influenza vaccines or we do not. Both heretical and orthodox expertise here relies on the same doxa for its rationale, despite the fact that the conclusions lead to distinct (in)action. Both heretics and orthodox often argue, then, that the other group does not understand the *basic science* of influenza. This underlying tension often came up in my conversation with representatives of both points of view. What follows is Fred Leung's response to a point that I had heard many times in my conversations with influenza experts, that flu viruses are inherently unpredictable.

> FL: No. This is wrong. Flu is unpredictable only because they don't understand the basic science. Most people get the virus mixed up. Even H1N1. This is the reason why everybody predicted that in the second wave, a hundred million people would die, and it didn't happen.
>
>   And how many people predict H5N1 will break out? For thirteen years we've been waiting for H5. And now, after thirteen years, when I go to a conference and say, "You don't need to kill all the chickens," I have fewer people throwing eggs at me, and starting to think that, yeah, maybe it makes sense. Because not just the laypeople misunderstood the virus. Scientists misunderstood the virus. See, most people don't understand mutation.

The virus is mutating every day, every second, by itself. The difference is, whether that mutation is driven or not.

TM: Wait, I don't quite understand. What do you mean?

FL: If you use vaccine, you drive mutation. If you don't use vaccine, you will, in some way, just let the natural host take care of the mutation rate.

When it concerns cross-species, whether a virus successfully establishes itself in the new host can only be understood by looking at the natural rules of how that virus works. We'll use SARS as an example, OK? SARS happened naturally, in that the coronavirus crossed over from animal into human. SARS is endemic in its host population. We learned from SARS that all you need to do when it crosses over is to lower the infection rate to less than one and the virus will eventually burn itself out. The more virulent the virus, the faster the virus dies out. By evolutionary principle. Before there is time to develop or use a vaccine. So, if you look at all the basic facts, and it is not that hard, you can bring the fear level down. The problem I have is that the world and the media and the politicians love to ramp that fear up. For whatever reason.

Today there are more BSL-3 labs and no money to sustain them all. Now, is that a wise decision? I don't think so. The WHO funded all these surveillance labs, in Indonesia, in Thailand, with unspoken rules that any data, anything that comes out, only the WHO can publish. Not the local scientists. If they somehow play the game, their names can be listed as co-authors. But you don't see that in the contract. You don't see that in the policy. But if you talk to the local scientists, that's what happened in practice. What drove Indonesians to refuse to share [H5N1 virus] samples? I'm not commenting on whether it is politically or ethically correct or not. But if you look at how influenza vaccines in particular are produced—the whole thing about vaccines and vaccine companies—their relationship with the CDC and the WHO and those agency's recommendations. I tell you, if it's not like a mafia, then what is it like?

Here we see a heretic directly questioning the foundation of the reigning influenza research paradigm—but not the need for research on influenza itself. Leung's critique of the orthodoxy is threefold: first, he troubles the current focus upon the development and manufacture of influenza vaccines and advocates for a more "basic" research program that would aid in the greater understanding of the virus's "natural" habits, its ecology; second, he problematizes the construction and maintenance of higher-level bios-ecurity labs in order to highlight the politics and fear-mongering that drive the demand for them; and finally, he suggests that the CDC and the WHO collude to produce a mafia—or unequal power structure that blocks others from effectively performing research on influenza. This type of critique is, in itself, part of a larger heretical narrative that unfurled during the play of events that were collectively referred to as the 2009 H1N1 pandemic.

At a biosecurity workshop I attended in the midst of the 2009 pandemic, I heard a similar refrain about the difficult and strained relationship be-tween health policy and epidemiological science from internationally re-spected virologist Adel Mahmoud. Mahmoud's own scientific research has been instrumental in the development of four vaccines for infectious diseases caused by viruses. For years before his retirement, he directed vac-cine research for a major pharmaceutical company. And yet in July 2009, he echoed Fred Leung's concern about the push to find a universal vaccine for every disease. The real danger, in Mahmoud's opinion, was the devel-opment over the decades of a type of "group think" within public health circles that had drifted toward "conservatism." When I asked him to talk a bit about public health's fascination with and reliance upon the almost mythical idea of a "vaccine," he responded with a lengthy discussion of the relationship between humans, microbes, science, and policy:

> *AM:* We as a community in general are fascinated by the idea of the magic bullet. That there is a single solution that will solve one— or more than one—of our problems. And that magic bullet is the most *absurd* concept—because most problems need an inte-grated, multifaceted approach to solve them.
>
> *TM:* How do we shift from that perspective, when it's been perceived as so successful in the past?
>
> *AM:* It has failed every time it was applied. Give me *one* example that it succeeded. The only odd example of a magic bullet that helped with one problem is the smallpox eradication with a vaccine. But since the mid-seventies, or the early seventies when we eradi-cated smallpox, to this date, we have gone after eradication as a concept. For many diseases. And we failed *every* time. We have been chasing polio now for the last nine years. It was supposed to

be 2000, 2002, 2005 . . . now they've stopped talking when. And I don't think it's going to be doable. You're chasing mirages!

So this fascination with the technical magic bullet solution, it's an easy thing to hang your hopes on. But it is amazingly, *amazingly*, short-sighted. And it has consistently failed. The subject matter of diseases is human populations. And human populations are not machines. They are social, they are cultural, they are economic, they are anthropological.

There was a serendipity to the discovery of smallpox vaccine. Since then, eighteen out of thirty vaccines still use the entire organism. So how much progress have we made since 1791? Our understanding of immunity mechanisms is close to zero. We are unable to discover what is an immunogen (with flu, as well as HIV and TB). The immunogen is not the H protein and we have to use the entire organism in vaccines.

With pandemic influenza? We've spent $8 billion, what do we have to show for it? There hasn't really been any progress vis-à-vis new vaccines, better vaccines, universal vaccines, etcetera. Without an increased understanding of these microbes and our response to them, we will not be able to make any new discoveries. Policy needs to be based on basic science. But innovation and discovery takes time. There is a great need for ecological and environmental understanding of microbes.

It's hilarious that there's this new emphasis on biological threats, since they've been with us forever. What are we going to do about the relationship between humans and microbes? Microbes are trying to self-defend. We need to change the war metaphor. In most cases, the relationship between microbes and humans is commensurate or symbiotic, and in a minimum of cases, it is pathological. To reduce our relationship to microbes to the anthrax attacks of 2001 is very sad. This is a philosophical mistake in policy making—reducing the interaction between us and microbes to post-9/11 thinking. Scare tactics never work because they only last for a certain amount of time and then they require another scare tactic.

Mahmoud is, in many ways, the perfect heretic. For many years, his research was at the center of both evolutionary virology and vaccine development. Mahmoud's heretical viewpoint, as that of a respected scientist and acknowledged expert, highlights how microbes such as the influenza virus continue to lie at the center of scientific expertise. The idea of studying viruses is not questioned within this narrative, but the utilization of the products of such research and the interpretation of knowledge about viruses such as Influenza A is troubled. At stake is whose expertise counts as the "correct" position on microbes. Of course, it should be noted here that Mahmoud's opinions above dovetail with my own. I remain partial to the heretical viewpoint that influenza is about more than just science and microbes. The problem of influenza is, clearly, also political and anthropological. But I agree, too, with the notion that disease surveillance is a "good" practice and I am also susceptible to the notion that studying viruses can tell us something more both about how they work and about how we understand ourselves in relationship to them.

The practice of studying viruses is never contested, then, by either side, even if vaccine technology is. Bowker and Star argue that "When an object becomes naturalized in more than one community of practice, its naturalization gains enormous power to the extent that a basis is formed for dissent to be viewed as madness or heresy" (1999, 312). Vaccines are such objects. The search for and development of vaccines is a cornerstone of epidemiology and public health practices, and has been ever since Edward Jenner "accidentally" discovered the smallpox vaccine. Neither Mahmoud nor Leung express a desire to do away entirely with vaccines, especially since they work to promote herd immunity. Rather, their attack is more subtle and exposes a "harmony of illusions" about the overall effectiveness of vaccines. Contradictions to the reigning thought style about vaccines are either "kept secret" or are the catalyst for "laborious efforts" to explain the exception, (Fleck 1979, 27.)

The interesting thing is that both Leung and Mahmoud partially explain their exceptional viewpoints through explication of their lives as experts on viruses, evolutionary virology, and the ecological aspects of viral life. These men see themselves as intimately connected to viruses. They have, in some ways, lived with them for decades. In everyday conversation, both men anthropomorphized viruses and talked about their relationship to the viruses they study as a natural part of their research lives. They understand viruses, then, because they have lived with them in their laboratories, become acquainted with their "natural habits," and spent countless hours working both with and on them, and ultimately learning from them.

Of course, orthodox experts feel much the same way. I often heard those working within the standard paradigms of influenza science and vaccine development talk about their own relationships to these invisible microbes in exactly the same way, framed as an integral part of their identities. Both heretical and orthodox experts consistently aver that they are "flu people" or "influenza people." This self-identification binds them together as much as does their collective research on influenza. Praxis—routine lab work on viruses—has given birth to a particular doxa about influenza. Next, I briefly explore the orthodoxy and its particularly charismatic narrative about the need for epidemiology to halt global outbreaks such as the 2009 H1N1 pandemic.

Charisma, Faith, and Doubt in the Orthodox Cathedral

The CDC's main auditorium was packed. Rohit pointed out important people in the audience, a Who's Who of public health experts. Near the podium on the stage at the front of the room stood William Foege, the speaker. As a former CDC director and a key figure in the fight to eradicate smallpox, Foege is a legendary figure not only at the CDC but within global public health, which accounted for the high turnout to hear his guest lecture.

The current director of the agency, Tom Frieden, introduced Foege by telling the audience that the lecture was taking place on the anniversary of the diagnosis of the final case of smallpox—exactly thirty-two years ago to the day. But because there was a waiting period of two years before the world could be officially declared "smallpox-free," we were officially celebrating the thirtieth anniversary of the eradication of smallpox. Foege, then, was part of a pivotal moment in the modern myth of public health— a lionized figure from a heroic past, when dominance over disease was still deemed a feasible dream, an achievable goal.

Indeed, the director's introduction to Foege's talk made no bones about this. Frieden told the audience that he had learned the following lesson from Foege: "Irrational optimism is a prerequisite for success in public health." Quoting Foege, Frieden went on to argue that surprise at success was an inappropriate response; it indicated a lack of faith in one's project. He argued that Foege was integral to global public health's commitment to the notion that methods and ideas should always be reevaluated in order to make them better.

From what I had observed, this was largely true. The very fact that any national health agency had allowed me into the heart of their operations was evidence enough of that. As was the director of the Global Disease Detection Program's request to hear my research findings and suggestions for improving the GDDOC's operation.

Foege began to speak. He was tall, imposing, elegant, and very handsome for his years. He had a white beard, glasses, a dark suit. He was all authority and wit and warmth. As a speaker, he was formidable. He peppered his talk with quotes from ancient Greece, from philosophers, from literature.

I was impressed and then, slowly and perceptibly, charmed by him. I could feel my natural skepticism sliding off as he talked and I listened, more and more enraptured. I had an urge to say something inappropriate to break the spell and I remembered having the same feeling sitting in a Catholic mass in Boston with my father on Easter Sunday. I realized that I was now sitting in a cathedral of public health. The tenor and message of public health was very missionary-like. I wasn't at a lecture; I was at a revival meeting. Foege was not a speaker; he was an archbishop.

Suddenly, I felt like a heretic myself. I had my yellow legal pad out, taking notes. I was a spy, an intruder, a *nonbeliever* in the cathedral.

Basically, I felt the same need to puncture the belief system—the groupthink—that was so palpably present in the room. I wanted everyone to know that I did not quite buy into all the "saving humanity from pestilence" business. I wanted to ask someone about the de facto authority and power that come along with science and public health.

But then, it was all so seductive.

There was also a part of me that liked the feeling of authority, that was all too comfortable working in a national health agency. There was a part of me that liked the fatherly man speaking. I wanted Foege to be right at the same time that I wanted to resist what he was saying in order to better hold it up for examination.

Foege told the audience he wanted to begin in the past and finish in the future. That this was what public health was about—learning from the past to help create a better future. I became more convinced about this being a missionary endeavor after he said, "No one ever leaves the CDC; they just become a CDC person in another location."

His talk jumped around from topic to topic. It sounded extemporane-ous and was completely nonlinear, but because he was such a command-ing presence, no one seemed to notice or to care. He started out talking about the last case of smallpox in Somalia. Then he moved on to mention the difference between international and global public health. This is a key point to understanding the ethics of public health. Foege asserted that the term "international" immediately brought up a dichotomy—pitting international health against its national counterparts. The term "global," however, transformed an outbreak anywhere into a local issue. The use of "global" asserted some kind of "natural right" to intervene—on behalf of global—not national—health. It sutured a fractured world back into what could be conceived of as a "global body" that needed to be protected against emerging infections.

It was a clever argument, and it was interesting that Foege seemed well aware of the import of word choice here. His use of "global" was no accident—it wasn't just a reaction to the so-called forces of globalization. It was purposeful in its intent to encompass the whole world as public health's domain and territory.

Foege called the CDC a "Gandhian" institution. But, Foege argued, the CDC had to re-earn the "Gandhi-an" label afresh each and every day— through science, the dispersal of that science, and through the way that members of the agency treated others. He argued that institutions—like people—could be mentors, and that the CDC had "molded" the thousands of people who had been trained there.

In essence, then, he was proselytizing. He told a story about being in India when the government announced that it had decided to rename its national public health agency to the National Centre for Disease Control. And just like that, a new branch of the church was born, joining others— the European Centre for Disease Prevention and Control, the Chinese Center for Disease Control—all modeled on the one, original CDC. There was more than branding at stake here; this was not just about a shared or-ganizational structure or shared methods, but about shared beliefs. People learned the craft of epidemiological science at the US CDC, and were then sent out in missionary style to other places to seed other churches of science.

Foege then said two things in close succession that puzzled me when taken together at face value. First, he said that "If you believed in fate, you wouldn't work here." Epidemiologists, he argued, could not afford to be "fainthearted" or "fatalistic." They must instead be bold enough to forge their own worlds. However, he then went on to suggest that public health workers must never be discouraged by the slow progress of their work. He told the audience: "Be assured of your contributions, even if you can't see them." These were slightly contradictory statements. Wasn't Foege asking his followers to be somewhat "fatalistic" in their belief that their contributions and efforts would eventually prevail? That the ultimate "fate" of public health was to succeed? Faith can make the idea of direct intervention seem untenable, yet the CDC as an institution is premised on the positive effects of such intervention.

Foege then likened the belief that the efforts of public health will ultimately be successful to the faith of those who built the medieval cathedrals. Architects and artisans in the Middle Ages would never live to see their creations built, but they had faith that the cathedrals they had planned and devoted their lives to erecting would *eventually* be built according to their best plans.

It was at this moment that I asked myself: Is the US CDC itself the Vatican of Global Public Health? Is the architecture of the CDC—of Buildings 1 through 26—the artifact of a set of past beliefs, of a certain type of faith in science to save the world? And what, if anything, would be able to shake that collective faith?

In his conclusion, Foege suggested that in the future, public health should encompass any and all determinants of health—including social and cultural factors. In other words, there was no limit to public health's territory, its domain of potential control and guidance. I found myself sitting in the audience thinking about biopower, life and death and their relationship, the future of government and its relationship to the new focus on global health. Just as I was pondering these things, Foege asserted that health was entirely incompatible with the marketplace and that capitalism was dangerous to health. In the past, he reminisced, "They told us to look over our shoulder for the socialists, but we never looked over our shoulder for the capitalists."

For his closing remark, he said that "I take comfort that H1N1 is being addressed by the CDC, and not Congress or the marketplace."

He received a standing ovation that lasted five minutes.

Expertise, Charisma, and the Production of Scientific Knowledge

To conclude, I argue here that Fred Leung's role throughout this chapter as a disbeliever in the narrative of catastrophic influenza pandemics and Adel Mahmoud's role as a questioner of rote vaccine development are together constitutive of the emergent character of the "heretic expert" in microbiology. As anthropologist Xin Liu has suggested: "Characters do not exist in isolation. There is always a set of characters whose full meaning can only be understood in relation to each other at a given historical moment" (2002, 24). For Liu, characters are distinct from the concept of "roles" in that characters are archetypes, generally understood as ideal types and thus useful in narrating a conception of the social world. I use the concept of the heretic as just such a character. It is only by looking at the heretic that the beliefs of the orthodox can be clearly discerned The debate between orthodox and heretic experts on the real threat of influenza is thus paradigmatic of how a virus has come to symbolize risk and preparedness in global public health over the past century.

Reading heretical and orthodox accounts juxtaposed, however, helps us to see how the narrative of influenza and scientific expertise itself are continuously negotiated among individuals with differing opinions, status as experts, and beliefs about the threat posed by the influenza virus. As Bowker and Star argue: "The memory comes in the form not of true or false facts but of multifaceted stories open to interpretation" (1999, 256). The personal narratives of influenza experts here show how we partially interpret our world through the lens of the influenza virus. As I argued in the first chapter about networks of viral expertise, human cultures are—in one way or another—shaped by viral cultures. In turn, both heretics and orthodox play a role in how we interpret this culture. They shape each other's viewpoints and create categories of competing expertise. As Ludwik Fleck noted almost a century ago, any scientific expert "is already a specially molded individual who can no longer escape the bonds of tradition and of the collective, otherwise he would not be an expert" (Fleck 1979, 54). The doxa of influenza science binds heretics and orthodox together, even when they disagree over the episteme or knowledge produced under the reigning research paradigm.

All the individual accounts and encounters with the influenza virus examined here—and this insight could be expanded to other infectious disease agents for that matter—are ultimately about the production of knowledge and systems of belief. There is an underlying tension throughout this chapter between facts and beliefs, though scientific expertise is often marshaled in defense of both. In fact, at times it was hard for me to tease out which statements were "fact" and which were "personal opinion"—especially when I was listening to a particularly charismatic expert. Charisma produced a temporary state of agreement; its effects often lingered for days or weeks after an interview. In essence, I had to remind myself that there was no "right answer" to the question of influenza, no "correct method" for dealing with it. Expertise notwithstanding, facts and information had always to be reintegrated with their context (see chapter 6), their significance realigned with a changing physical and intellectual landscape. I had to rely on my own anthropological expertise to help me sort out what the 2009 H1N1 pandemic meant without falling back into the trap of "not if, but when"–style thinking myself.

Scientific research must be interpreted (as we saw in chapter 6) for it to have meaning. Debates and disagreements over the meaning of influenza and the 2009 H1N1 pandemic are negotiated to produce a narrative of events. However, those interpretations are highly volatile and continuously being renegotiated. Historians wait decades after an event is over to examine it because the stories are still shifting. Anthropologists, sociologists, and political scientists cannot be that circumspect. Rather, we must dive into the meaning-making pool while the narratives are yet being crafted. And so, this book ends with the personal tales not only of my informants, but of my own relationship to events in 2009. Pathography is not a tidy technique, but it is a necessary one for understanding disease events on a global scale.

EPILOGUE

Gene Segment NS. Biological Function: *NS1 is a nonstructural virus poly-peptide that is thought to interfere with a host's immune response. Changes in the genetic makeup of this segment are hypothesized to be directly related to Influenza A viruses' pathogenicity. In particular, H5N1's NS segment is thought to be a direct cause of its virulence. The 1918 H1N1 virus's NS1 segment is surmised to be at the root of its infamous degree of pathogenicity. Because of this, the NS gene segment is a target of universal Influenza A vac-cine development for both humans and birds. NS2 codes for a nuclear export protein that aids in the process of viral transcription.* Pathographic Function: *This final segment examines why narratives of an influenza pandemic remain so culturally persuasive—or virulent—and how the concept of pathography might prove a useful tool in understanding future outbreaks of novel influenza viruses. In essence, then, this segment is a bridge to future social-scientific stud-ies of outbreaks, pandemics, other health "crises," and pathogenic happenings on a global scale.*

A Tale of Multiple Viruses

As I was finishing this book, in late December 2013, narratives of influenza continued unabated. On December 20, the WHO issued a routine influenza report indicating that the flu season in North America was beginning to pick up its pace. The influenza virus in circulation was A(H1N1) pdm09—or the same virus at the heart of this pathography. In fact, two early-season clusters of cases in Texas had been particularly severe, killing four of those infected and drawing renewed attention to the 2009 H1N1 virus. The prodigal virus, given enough time, always seems to return.

By the start of 2014, a diverse family of avian influenza viruses appeared poised to continue our story in novel and curious ways. The WHO had officially confirmed two new cases of H7N9 in China and local and global experts were continuing to closely monitor the situation as it developed. Cases of H7N9 had sporadically appeared since the novel virus's first appearance in humans in March; each one triggered similar fears about the possibility of H7N9 mutating into a strain that could cause a deadly bird flu pandemic. But H7N9 was not the only Influenza A virus to jump the species divide from birds into humans in 2013. In Jianxi Province, China, another avian influenza virus, H10N8, had also been able to cross over, and infect and kill an elderly woman. And in neighboring Taiwan, a novel H6N1 virus (one similar in structure to H7N9) infected a young woman. A late December outbreak of an H5N2 virus at a poultry farm in China's Hebei Province drove authorities to slaughter 127,000 birds in an effort to contain the virus and prevent any human infections.

All things considered, by January 2014 it almost seemed as if influenza was mocking the experts who study it by continuing to defy all their expectations and predictive models. And while the flu continued to beguile and frustrate scientists and epidemiologists, the collective narratives concerning future pandemics persisted. In fact, the story of influenza is itself continually mutating in increasingly interesting and endless ways. There is something about the influenza virus that almost compels our collective imaginations and attempts at preemptive public health actions. Viruses like influenza are invisible co-inhabitors of our planet. Perhaps the flu reminds us that we are all vulnerable, binding us together in our susceptibility. Or perhaps it's more complicated than that.

In 2012, two separate laboratories working on the H5N1 virus (both quite famous labs in flu circles) announced that they had been successful in efforts to genetically alter the virus, making it more transmissible between mammals. Here's the twist: instead of waiting for so-called natural changes to occur, or simply tracking evolutionary changes in the virus somewhere out in the "wild" where birds, pigs, and humans intermingled and swapped packets of RNA, these enterprising scientists had manipulated the virus in order to directly affect its transmissibility and severity. This, they argued, was the best way to learn how viruses worked. Not watching them in their natural habitats, but directly manipulating or mimicking possible evolutionary changes in the lab. In other words, the best way to study viruses might be to learn to "think" like them. Controversy over the safety of this research, a temporary moratorium on any further manipulation or publication of scientific results, and the development of new research guidelines as a result of this work all reconstructed the H5N1 virus as both a natural and a man-made threat.

Evolutionary virologists, like the ones in this book, sequence novel flu viruses that they collect during routine surveillance. They hope that by comparing and analyzing viral RNA, they can begin to better understand how influenza viruses evolve in their natural environments. These environments include, however, not only the lakes and ponds that wild birds frequent, but also animal farms and urban markets and all the places where humans and pigs and ducks and chickens come into close contact with each other. Which is, if you think about it, quite a lot of places (backyard chicken enclosures and state fairs included). In other words, the ecology of viruses is intimately mixed up with the ecology of humans. Our co-evolution is what I'm interested in here—how viral "reassortants" blur the lines between us and them, humans and birds and pigs, creating a "pandemic humanity"[1] that's all-encompassing—the focus of global health prevention programs writ large.

Reassortment works in two ways: either by the slow accrual of small genetic changes as viruses replicate (genetic drift) or by swapping segments with other viruses in a host (genetic shift). It's the bigger shifts—or reassortment events—that everyone in this book is ultimately worried about, and that are seen as having the potential to produce a "killer" virus. Evolutionary virologists hope that by learning about viral origins and interactions, a virus's "ecology," they can better predict the type of environments and interactions that lead to problematic admixtures of human and nonhuman. Reassortants are, in short, viruses that consist of parts from multiple species—they are mutant, hybrid, and not one thing or another but everything at once. They blur the lines between disparate things by being able to infect all of us. Epidemiologists and virologists think reassortants are dangerous to our health because none of us—birds, pigs, or humans—have natural immunity to such monstrous viral offspring. We are all susceptible; and it is this concept of universal susceptibility that in turn breeds a particular type of community. As Priscilla Wald has argued, contagion is "the color of belonging, social as well as biological" (2008, 12). Viruses like H5N1—or the recent outbreaks of the novel H7N9 virus in China—suggest that birds and pigs and humans and other infectable mammals actually "belong" to the same "herd" populations (at least from the perspective of the viruses that infect us). And since these viruses have the ability to infect everyone, they also blur national and cultural and social and political and economic boundaries between human populations. As any epidemiologist can tell you, in order to protect someone somewhere, you have to protect everyone everywhere. It is the formation of what I will refer to as a universal body in need of protection or a "pandemic humanity" in relationship to bird flu that I want to focus on here.

The scientific practices that center on understanding how viruses evolve engender the concept of pandemic humanity on multiple levels. Reassortant events—the births of new viruses—highlight the flows of multiple objects—viruses, birds, soil samples, scientific techniques, data, RNA segments, chicken breasts—that constitute the "ecology" of both bird flu and the humans that they infect. And "who" they can infect is, well, everyone. As Starr and Griesemer argue about the usage of ecology within the framework of both science and social science: "The important questions concern the flow of objects and concepts through the network of participating allies and social worlds. The ecological viewpoint is antireductionist" (507). To borrow from Dominic Boyer's recent work on informational ecology, I argue that in the world of avian influenza research, surveillance, and prevention the scientific paradigm "has been overwhelmed by and absorbed into 'the environment'"(Boyer 2013, 170). Viral ecology has no natural limits because husbandry practices are implicated in the "natural" evolution of "wild" viruses. In evolutionary virology, the habitats of avian influenza viruses are boundless and constantly in motion. Global flows[2] are viral flows, and the distinctions between them are very hard to tease out.

The bodies at risk here are at once human and nonhuman; the real and imagined risk of exposure to avian influenza viruses helps to construct a pandemic humanity that is always already materially interconnected with its "environment." Even a concept like "exposure" in the realm of the pandemic human is complicated. Exactly who is being exposed to whom? Pigs are exposed to ducks; chickens are exposed to humans; ducks are exposed to chickens; humans are exposed to pigs; pigs are exposed to humans. All of us are exposed to viruses. Reassortant viruses cannot exist, cannot function, without each of us. We produce them and they infect us in a never-ending loop. The material world—farms, fences, migratory routes, lakes, duck feces (this is a huge focus of scientific research, by the way, as chicken and duck feces are where most researchers find their best viruses)—is an integral part of the cycle. But forget Latour's actor-network theory (2005) for helping to untangle this mess—we would all be in the field forever, endlessly tracing all the associations and flows and practices until we dropped dead from exhaustion. Exposure to viruses makes our normal, everyday environments inherently risky. Indeed, the very word conjures up notions of risk and uncertainty and susceptibility. Viruses like H7N9 reflect an emergent awareness that we are all impossibly entangled—both genetically and otherwise—with the worlds around us. Influenza viruses work to create and undergird pandemic humanity.

Although the concept as I deploy it here relies upon the construction of a global population that is both susceptible and in need of care, pandemic humanity is not necessarily about the creation of a new type of global or "pandemic" biopower. Biopower, as Foucault formulated it, takes the individual human body first as a machine to be disciplined and then as a species body that must be regulated (1973). In relationship to governmentality, the individual qua family morphs into a (self-)governable population at the same time that economy is inserted into politics (Foucault 1979). The "body" under biopower and governmentality, or biopolitics, is an object for discipline, control, and regulation—collectively forming a body politic that is fully contained in an intricate web of state power. But pandemic humanity conjures a different type of hybrid body; reassortants necessarily mutate our conceptions about the human body and its relationship to things like viruses and chickens, and thus, in the process, begins to alter the very concept of biopower itself. While the admonitions to cover your mouth, wash your hands, get a flu shot, and so forth, seem to fall squarely under the biopolitical rubric of "self-care" (Foucault 1988), the myriad human (and nonhuman) practices that make up our viral "ecology" don't fit neatly into biopolitical analyses of disease. Biopolitics relies upon a conception of a sovereign body being attacked from without and within (see Esposito 2008 for an examination of the "immunity paradigm" in relationship to a reimagining of the concept of biopolitics in the twenty-first century). But the body within pandemic humanity is anything but a self-contained fortress forever in need of discipline, regulation, and defense. Viruses, as any virologist will tell you, are not so easily controlled or contained or easy to separate out from their hosts; they reassort or not, seemingly at will and at serendipitous times and places ostensibly of their own choosing.

What reassortant viruses teach us, then, is that we live in an interconnected (or networked), global, and viral world. In essence, what I want to provocatively suggest is that *the global is viral*. I mean this in two registers. First, like a biological virus, the global cannot exist outside of a host. There is no "global" without "local" institutions, structures, agencies, and individuals. Second, like a computer virus, the global is constituted by information that moves and flows and mutates and self-replicates. This pathography began as an attempt to show how a global pandemic operated; it ends by highlighting, in part, just why anything "global" is often so hard to pin down and any "thing" or event that is global in scope or scale can initially seem impossible to study effectively (think of international finance or international relations, as just two equally pernicious examples). Globally circulating viruses like H1N1, H5N1, or H7N9 simply highlight all the ways in which the boundaries between living and nonliving, human and nonhuman, us and them are artificially constructed and have—quite frankly—been dangerous to our health.

Thinking about these viruses should make us ask some interesting—and unanswered—questions: Which reassortants are more dangerous? The ones that evolve "naturally" or the ones that are "manmade"—and more importantly—can we really tell the difference? Is there one? Which viruses should we be worried about? What is pandemic humanity's risk or susceptibility and how is the concept being used to undergird the daily functioning and raison d'être of an emergent global public health? How might understanding the ecology of influenza viruses mess with our notions about who and what we are?

A long time ago I wrote a paper about the possible philosophical effects of the then new discovery that our own DNA is made up of quite a bit of leftover viruses (MacPhail 2004). In essence, I argued, as I did in the

introduction of this book, that humans are just a conglomeration of viruses with shoes. The focus on viral ecology and the scientific and popular
reimagining of life along viral lines (see Zimmer 2012) is merely a reflection of the fact that we have always been "reassortants." Trying to write a
pathography of pandemic humanity is then, in many ways, simply doing
anthropology for the twenty-first century.

An Ending of No Ending

This pathography is perforce an unfinished narrative. Initially conceived
as an examination of the myth of a killer avian influenza pandemic and our
collective fascination with deadly viruses, it has ended up as an analysis of
the very real events that unfolded near the start of my fieldwork in 2009.
What started *in medias res* must then end there, too. How could there be an
end to the story of an influenza virus like H1N1 or H5N1, especially one
so recent in linear history that its narratives are constantly being rewritten,
reshaped, and retold? And when subsequent narratives tied into the 2009
pandemic, such as the ones briefly alluded to above, are themselves still
unfolding?

As I argued at the beginning of this book, there is no one "story" of the
2009 H1N1 influenza pandemic. Rather, the various accounts of the events
that took place in 2009—including this one—are part of a much larger
metanarrative about influenza and about pandemics themselves. To echo
one of the pioneers of information technology, sociologist Ted Nelson, everything about influenza is "intertwingled." Such being the case, this has
been my attempt to gather as many of those intertwinglings as possible in
order to recreate a three-dimensional picture of what a pandemic is, what
influenza and information about influenza do, and what it means to be an
expert producing knowledge within global public health today.

Regular narratives and methods do not work well when we are analyzing anything global or virtual or assembled or multiple such as outbreaks
of infectious diseases. Things like a global pandemic require us, as social
scientists, to invent new means or to modify old tools in order to grapple
with them. Pathography in the traditional sense is simply a medical narrative of the progression of an illness in a particular patient. As such, it tries
to understand something about the disease itself through its expression

in the individual. Like ethnography, it interests itself in the particular in order to understand something greater about the universal. In its literary sense, pathography is the term used to describe memoirs or biographies that focus upon of all the negative events in a single life that have affected its subject. Similar to medical narratives, a literary pathography tries to take an individual's lived experience and connect it back into the collective human experience. It is the effort to reconnect and to make sense of one's own narrative that makes such memoirs particularly compelling. My usage here attempts to straddle both of these usages by combining it with traditional ethnography. Global public health and pandemic humanity are thus conceptualized as superorganic subjects that both became infected with influenza.

Near the beginning of this project, and especially while working inside the CDC in a unit whose job it is to keep track of international outbreaks and to gather and share information with partner agencies around the world, I often found myself wondering what was "global" about global public health in the first place. The "global" has been an object of concern for anthropologists and other social scientists from at least the 1980s onward. In the post–World War II period, the spread of capitalism (and other "Western" structures and ideas) spurred an increased interest in and awareness of the various practices and policies that have come to define "globalization" or "neoliberalism." I would like to conclude this pathography by arguing that the "global" in global public health reflects a reimaging of the concept itself. By the end of my fieldwork, I realized that global public health is as viral as the viruses it tracks, collects, studies, reproduces, manipulates, and helps to contain or eradicate.

The "global" in relationship to public health reflects that we are not only living in a virosphere (or a world dominated by viruses), but in the epoch of the Anthropocene (or a world dominated by human viruses). If things that are "global" are necessarily viral by nature, and I would argue that they are, then pathography is a perfect tool for unpacking them. Pathography lets us pay closer attention to the way things—narratives, actors, objects—are interconnected. As a methodology, pathography lingers with the virgule in the following stubborn dualities: macro/micro, local/global, subject/object, nature/culture, knowledge/belief, science/society, past/future. The symbol of the global as viral is the "/" that connects these concepts. The viral traffics in these social and cultural dichotomies without necessarily reifying them. The way in which the chapters of this book moved from the micro to the macro, from Hong Kong to Atlanta, from the lab to the WHO, from the past to the future and back again has, in essence, been an attempt to interweave genes and memes in order to go beyond these categorizations or binaries.

The chapters of this book on biology, history, geography, narratives, information, and the lab should be read together as an ethnography of the everyday practices that occur *during* a historic event. Focusing either on "events" or on the "everyday" too often creates a false dichotomy that is not necessarily experienced by those living through, as the Chinese malediction goes, such "interesting times." From the standpoint of the experts I knew, the everyday of a microbiology lab or a public health institution simply folded into the year-long pandemic; in 2009, the boundaries between the everyday and the event blurred to the point of abstraction. The everyday became a part of the crisis and then the crisis became part of the everyday. Indeed, and as scholar Lauren Berlant has recently argued, the modern era is one of persistent crisis or uncertainty, wherein the experience of the 2009 pandemic might be better described as a "crisis ordinary" (Berlant, 9), or an unfolding series of events. In a crisis ordinary, our everyday, lived experiences, events are not always memorable; rather, they are "*episodes*, that is, occasions that frame experience while not changing much of anything" (Berlant 2011, 101). The various narratives about "bird flu" or influenza within this book are pertinent examples of the ordinary, and somewhat permanent, crises that continue to unfold without end.

NOTES

Prologue to a Pathography

1. While I expect that pathography as a concept and method will be most useful to fellow medical anthropologists, sociologists, historians, and science studies scholars who research illness, disease, or the biological sciences, I think that it might also be useful to the examination and analysis of other negative events—such as the financial crisis, mass shootings, or natural disasters.

2. Pandemics are not abnormal in the sense that they occur every year in the normal flu season, typically from October to May in the Northern Hemisphere. Though we associate the term "pandemic" with a severe outbreak of disease—such as those seen in movies such as *Outbreak* and *Contagion*—most pandemics of influenza are much milder in nature and technically happen on a regular basis. Because of this, the WHO created pandemic threat levels to aid public health practitioners in planning more effectively for different scales of pandemic response. The system came under attack as a result of the 2009 H1N1 pandemic, leading to an ongoing reevaluation of the threat level system's overall usefulness.

3. Currently, there are seventeen known subtypes of HA and ten of NA, whose combinations produce different viral strains that cause varying severity of disease. The Influenza A viruses at the center of this pathography, H1N1 and H5N1, are named for their HA and NA subtypes.

4. There are some vocal exceptions to this consensus. I will explore the views of these dissenters in chapter 7.

5. A detailed examination of this shift in thinking about the value of junk DNA and viruses in the genome, as well as its larger philosophical implications in regard to the relationship between life and death, can be found in MacPhail 2004.

6. I am indebted to my friend (and molecular biologist) Matthew Lawlor for suggesting this term.

7. In contrast to the use of similar terms in earlier works (Durkheim 1984 [1893], Kroeber 1917, Spencer 1969 [1876]), I expand on Nicholas Christakis's conception of the superorganism as an assemblage of individuals in a network. A network for Christakis is something more than the sum of its individuals; the network aggregates and distributes knowledge and creates value in the form of social capital (2010). This is not to argue, however, that the network I'm describing here is "organic" in Durkheim's usage of the term, or that it takes primacy over the individuals who comprise it. Unlike more familiar terms often deployed by social scientists to describe the connections between people and things, such as "assemblage" or "network," a superorganism in my usage here is an *organism*.

A brief note here on the difference between the superorganism as a "network of networks" and the network as it has been conceptualized in prior research in the social sciences (see Latour 2005 and Riles 2000 for two exemplars of recent work that deploys the network as a generative analytical tool). While a "network" in common parlance can be scaled up or down and consists of as few as a handful of individuals or as many as hundreds of persons and/or objects, the superorganism operates at a "metalevel" of analysis. It is an aggregate of other networks big and small. In the case of the 2009 H1N1 pandemic, the superorganism of global public health had no "center" and consisted of many other, smaller, networks. The superorganism emerges or fades away in response to a large event or a crisis; it is thus "temporary," but in its creation of stronger bonds between its networks, each reemergence of the superorganism in response to a similar event will be that much easier and faster. The superorganism's makeup is constantly shifting and continuously needs to be remade and maintained. And yet, as a whole, it has capabilities for collective sense-making, knowledge production, and decision-making that do not exist at smaller scales. In Mary Douglas's terms, I understand a superorganism to be—akin to her usage of the term "institution" through Durkheim and Fleck—a "legitimized social grouping" (Douglas 1986, 46). Like institutions, superorganisms grant identity, classify things like viruses, can remember and forget events or facts, and are responsible for making life or death decisions on a grand scale.

1. Seeing the Past or Telling the Future?

1. A "naïve" population is one that has never been exposed to a particular influenza strain and thus has no in-built immunity to the virus. For example, most people have never been exposed to H5N1, and so the human immune system is ill-equipped to fend off infection. A virus such as H1N1 or H3N2 has circulated before in the general population. However, if it has changed enough, it will still be capable of evading an "experienced" immune system.

2. Robert Koch was one of the first microbiologists. Using his work on tuberculosis as a model, he formulated the criteria—called Koch's postulates—for determining if a particular microbe caused a disease or was merely an opportunistic co-infector. The organism must be found in the animal, must be capable of being isolated, must produce disease in a healthy animal, and must be recovered from the diseased animal.

3. Science often progresses through such examples of serendipity. Ferrets are still the preferred research animals for studying influenza—a preference that has its beginnings in this chance event. The controversy over H5N1 research in 2012 was over an engineered strain that was capable of spreading more easily from ferret to ferret than its "wild" (naturally occurring) counterparts.

4. Unfortunately, the science of vaccine development for influenza has had difficulty progressing past this initial breakthrough. The influenza virus does not grow well—or at all—in human cells, and seasonal vaccines are still manufactured using chicken eggs. However, because influenza kills chickens, it has been difficult to develop a vaccine for more virulent strains of influenza—such as H5N1. In recent years, the US government has been funding research into new methods for developing influenza vaccines. As of this printing, some of that research has

shown great promise. Research on a "universal" influenza vaccine—one that could be used no matter which strain is circulating—has also been progressing. There is renewed hope, in the light of these recent scientific advances, that influenza will no longer be a serious threat to human health in the foreseeable future.

5. In 2011, the WHO changed the name of GISN to the Global Influenza Surveillance and Response System (GISRS) following the adoption of its new Pandemic Influenza Preparedness (PIP) Framework.

6. For an overview of the shift from prevention to preparedness in public health, see Lakoff and Collier's *Biosecurity Interventions* (2008). For a review of the shift in national security in the United States, see Joe Masco's *The Theater of Operations: Affective Infrastructures of the National Security State* (forthcoming).

7. The United States has one of the largest intellectual, organizational, and financial commitments to this preparedness effort. As examples, see the Department of Homeland Security's National Strategy for Pandemic Influenza: Implementation Plan, and the Department of Health and Human Services' Pandemic Influenza Plan.

8. Most of the scientists and epidemiologists I worked with or interviewed during the pandemic still used "swine flu" as shorthand for the virus in informal conversations, well after the WHO had officially named the virus as *2009 A (H1N1) Influenza*. The renaming was due in part to better information about its genetic sequence and in part due to pushback from Mexico and complaints from the pork industry. In official communiqués, however, public health professionals were diligent about the use of the officially sanctioned scientific nomenclature, partially to avoid running into any more "cultural issues" related to the use of "swine flu."

9. When I asked a microbiologist to review this chapter, his reaction was as follows: "Mad Cow is a prion-based disease with no treatment and no cure that is transmitted by eating cooked food with prions in it. To my knowledge there is no evidence that the influenza virus could ever survive any type of cooking process (heck, even a marinade would probably sufficiently disrupt the virion structure). You should also mention Senator Grassley's infamous hearings where he called officials to testify just so they could state on TV that 2009 H1N1 is unrelated to eating pork."

10. Despite the fact that "definitive" answers to the question of a particular flu strain's origins—either in biological or geographical terms—are not possible to obtain, the search for them persists. I would like to point out here that both the lay and the expert desire to discover the origins of influenza viruses are socially constructed. The search for origins, however fruitless it may sometimes appear on the surface, provides a very real foundation for productive scientific research in evolutionary virology.

11. Almost immediately, the 2009 H1N1 virus was compared to the 1918 H1N1 virus. Scientists were on the lookout for any genetic markers or similarities to the 1918 strain that might indicate that the burgeoning pandemic would be deadlier than a "normal" flu strain. I will talk about this comparison in more detail in the section to follow.

12. Timely access to samples of novel or reemergent viruses is critical, and the sharing of virus samples—especially at the international level—can sometimes become a contentious topic. See MacPhail 2009 for an analysis of Indonesia's and China's reluctance to share samples of avian influenza viruses as one pertinent example. In the case of the 2009 H1N1 outbreak, the first available samples of the virus out of Mexico bypassed the CDC labs in Atlanta, and were shipped instead to Canada. This incident caused a few ruffled feathers inside the CDC, which had expected to be the first to receive samples from their counterpart agency in Mexico. I will touch on this topic again in a later chapter on data and information sharing, networks, and diplomacy in global public health.

13. The speed and efficiency of information sharing during the earliest days and weeks of the 2009 pandemic was the result of years of pandemic planning, attendant efforts to develop sophisticated IT programs and websites for information exchange, as well as collective efforts to

strengthen and build the global public health network (by running, as just one example, tabletop exercises that helped to increase familiarity and trust between different nodes).

14. Influenza viruses are unique in that they have been collected and studied "in different geographical regions" by scientists for well over a century, and thus provide a good "resource" for virologists interested in studying evolutionary change in RNA viruses (Webster et al. 1992). In fact, this rich, century-long data source is the reason that virologists Stephen Morse and Ann Schluederberg labeled influenza as a "model" for studying "viral emergence" writ large in their seminal article, "Emerging Viruses: The Evolution of Viruses and Viral Diseases" (1990). Many scholars have since linked our modern obsession with "emergent" viruses (think Nipah, Ebola, and Marburg) to this article, published in the *Journal of Infectious Diseases*.

15. I use "phylogeny" instead of "genealogy" here due, in part, to the ways in which researchers are both materially and discursively related. Phylogeny is, therefore, related to Foucault's concept of genealogy, but attends to the material ways in which virologists are connected (through viral samples, techniques, and material practices).

16. To borrow from science studies scholars Harry Collins and Robert Evans (2007), expertise in global public health is "real" not simply "relational" (2), even if attaining that expertise is a "social process" (3) as much as it is a scientific one. In other words, viral expertise is not simply the product of virologists and epidemiologists' relationships with each other. There is, Collins and Evans suggest, something substantive about expertise, grounded as it is in the daily production of scientific information about viruses. As such, it is both material and relational, embodied and discursive. What I have tried to highlight in this chapter is the ways in which an expert's past experience crafts and affects his expertise. In daily interactions with other scientists and with viruses in the lab, virologists and epidemiologists construct and reconfigure a larger "phylogeny of viral expertise" through their collective attempts to locate and understand the "origins" of pandemic Influenza A viruses. As Pierre Bourdieu suggests: "When [scientists] try to express their sense of correct procedure, they have little to call on beyond their past experience, which remains implicit and quasi-corporeal, and when they talk informally about their research, they describe it as a practice requiring experience, intuition, skill, flair, a 'knack,' all things difficult to set down on paper, which can only really be understood and acquired by example and through personal contact with competent persons" (2004, 39). It is within this context—or the milieu of influenza science—that expertise about flu is formed.

17. One might wonder here if the fact that both the 1918 and the 2009 pandemic influenza strains were H1N1 led those familiar with events early in the last century to react more forcefully and fearfully to the initial outbreak. "Better safe than sorry" was the collective mantra of all the flu experts I came into contact with throughout the second wave of the pandemic. The rationale for acting quickly to declare a pandemic was certainly not separate from the anxiety over the potential for the 2009 H1N1 strain to act more like it's deadlier "cousin."

18. The cost effectiveness of sequencing has changed dramatically since 2009. It is now less costly, making sequencing entire genomes more feasible.

19. For a detailed description of the lab practices and processes that turn soil samples into information on influenza, see chapter 2.

2. The Invisible Chapter (Work In the Lab)

1. An important note on the effect of technology on the production of knowledge within the lab: While the basic processes and procedures for obtaining genetic information from viral samples are largely uniform, the equipment—and thus the set of techniques—often differs depending on the funding level of each lab. Dr. Leung's lab used slightly "older" technology, so the descriptions that follow may seem outdated to anyone using newer technologies to produce genetic information.

2. The scientists who reviewed this chapter often commented upon just how much ennui they experienced in the lab. One reviewer even suggested I change the phrasing here from "surprising" silences to "often oppressive."

3. "Wet labs" is the term used to refer to laboratories that deal with biological materials. "Dry labs" are biological labs that do not deal with "wet" material, but with the "dry" information about them. Typically, dry labs utilize the information produced in wet labs.

4. Should an anomaly occur at any stage of the process, or if something should happen outside of standard lab protocol, Raymond would create a record of it in order to relate the anomaly to the end result.

5. For an interesting exploration of the separation of mind and body in relationship to the production of intellectual work and the phenomenology of expertise, see Dominic Boyer's article on the "corporeality of expertise" (2005).

6. For an example of how the development of PCR utterly transformed how scientific knowledge is produced, see Rabinow 1996.

3. Quarantine, Epidemiological Knowledge, and Infectious Disease Research in Hong Kong

1. When I sent an earlier version of this chapter to Ben Cowling for review, he pointed out that 132 is the number of lab-confirmed cases only. A paper co-authored by Cowling and recently published in the *Lancet* reported that perhaps as many as 27,000 infections of H7N9 have occurred (Yu et al. 2013). See the article for a full scientific assessment of the virus's clinical severity.

2. Past pandemics, such as the one in 1957, did originate in China. Recent scientific findings suggest that influenza viruses are more easily transmissible under rainy and humid conditions (Tamerius et al. 2013), such as those found in southern China and Southeast Asia year-round.

3. For a detailed analysis of how "bird flu" became synonymous with H5N1 and was thus conceptualized as a "Chinese" virus, see MacPhail 2009.

4. Some Chinese farmers house chickens, ducks, and geese near pigs. Pigs have been suggested as "mixing vessels" for influenza viruses. Some scientists think that swine infected with multiple strains of influenza can provide a suitable environment for gene swapping, producing new viral reassortments. Since pigs have physical similarities to humans, such a deadly strain in a pig would be more likely than one originating in a bird to start a global pandemic of influenza in humans. The virologist Robert Webster is a staunch supporter of this idea.

5. My thanks to an anonymous reviewer for suggesting this turn of phrase. It fit so perfectly that I integrated it like a virus into the conceptual RNA of this book.

6. For a detailed historical account of how the concept of *weisheng* or hygiene was interpreted as a sign of Western modernity and Chinese inferiority by Chinese elites in Tianjin, China, see Rogaski 2004.

7. Disease here is located by the colonial administration within the Chinese body itself. The lived-in bodies of the Chinese are transformed, after death, into mere repositories of disease. The "Chinese body" here is instrumentalized through the medical gaze of Western researchers, stripped of all its social, economic, cultural, and gendered aspects in order to transform multiple bodies into a "blank" site for the study of bacteriology. Nancy Scheper-Hughes and Margaret Lock, in their article "The Mindful Body: A Prolegomenon to Future Work in Medical Anthropology" (1987), argue that there are in effect three distinct bodies: the individual body, with its attendant phenomenology; the social body, which is the domain of symbolic and structural anthropologies; and the political body, tied to poststructuralism and Foucauldian notions of biopower. In the rhetoric that constructs the Hong Kong body as a disease resource above, there is no easily locatable "individual" body—and no semblance of the embodied or "lived" experience of illness.

8. I should note here that the official response was not perfect. The infection figure of 1,700 cases was due to slow implementation of hospital infection control measures (ones that are now

standard throughout the SAR). The head of the Hospital Authority was fired as a result, and the leadership and decision-making of then Director of Health Margaret Chan was severely questioned. Indeed, Margaret Chan's reputation within Hong Kong, in spite of her later attainment of director generalship of the WHO, is not a fully positive one.

9. In 2003, infectious disease outbreaks were still classified by the Communist Chinese Party (CCP) as state secrets. Information related to outbreaks could thus only be officially disseminated by the CCP itself. The initial outbreak of SARS was reported to the international public health community by rogue doctors and epidemiologists working in China and initial information circulated as "rumor."

10. A concrete example of the inherent difficulty and slipperiness of Hong Kong's global position vis-à-vis public health was the election of Margaret Chan, a Hong Kong "native," as the first "Chinese" director general of the WHO. Chan was "constructed as a 'Chinese Hong Konger,' rather than an ordinary Chinese person" (Shen 2008, 362) by both the Hong Kong and the Chinese media throughout her campaign for the position. Her role in Hong Kong during the SARS crisis was a key factor in her election. The election of Chan marked a turning point in China–Hong Kong relations, as the first instance of a native Hong Konger being elected to represent the mainland at a high level of international diplomacy (Shen 2008, 364). Chan is trained in Western methods, but is Chinese in citizenship and in terms of her "culture." This type of "in-between-ness" made her the perfect "Chinese" representative for election to an international regulatory body. In essence, then, Chan—like Hong Kong itself—spanned the East/West divide and represented a new "Chineseness" on the world stage.

11. While the Hong Kong SAR arguably fits under the rubric of *postcoloniality* as a condition—it was indeed a British possession for over a century—the territory and its populace are not as easily captured through the lens of *postcolonialism* as a theory (for a clear differentiation of these closely related concepts, see Gandhi 1998). For one, and as highlighted throughout the earlier sections of this chapter, Hong Kong seems to have little overweening "desire to forget the colonial past" or "postcolonial amnesia." What is more, there is scant on-the-ground evidence that the local government is actively trying to "make a new start" post-handover. Hong Kong's long history of British, and now Chinese, rule highlights the ways in which the city and its denizens trouble the two postcolonial positions of "contestation and its discomfiting other, complicity." (Gandhi 1998, 4, 5.) Hong Kong does not need to be reminded of its colonial past, nor does it seem to need with to break with it. Rather, Hong Kong identifies as both/and as well as neither/nor.

12. It often seemed that no group was more surprised—or almost impishly delighted—that the 2009 H1N1 influenza virus had not sprung out of the Hong Kong SAR or Guangdong Province than the collection of flu experts working in the region. The SAR was familiar enough with being suspected as an "incubator" or epicenter of infectious disease outbreaks, such as SARS or avian influenza, but had scant experience with being on the furthest periphery of them. Most national pandemic flu plans rely upon a planning model that anticipates China as the origin point of most novel strains of influenza; thus most nations, excluding China, were primed to defend against the importation of disease—not its export. Hong Kong, on the other hand, is and was fully prepared to play both defense and offense against the virus.

13. Some infectious disease agents, such as Ebola, require close contact in order to spread. Quarantine is seen as a particularly effective tactic in such cases. The viruses that cause SARS and MERS also require relatively close contact, and so are thought to be susceptible to containment measures to contain their spread. Influenza, and other such highly contagious and easily spread diseases, is seen as being less affected by containment measures. For one, many such diseases have "healthy carriers" (people infected—and able to spread the disease—who show no symptoms) and/or late onset of symptoms (carriers of flu often shed viruses—or are highly contagious—well before they come down with any telltale symptoms such as fever or headache), making quarantine a far less effective response tactic. The length of containment time required to "catch" all cases would be a logistical nightmare for public health authorities.

4. The Siren's Song of Avian Influenza

1. A number of flu experts believe the morbidity and mortality of the 1918 pandemic was primarily due to secondary infections of bacterial pneumonia. As such, these experts suggest that modern antibiotics and improved hygiene make another equally deadly pandemic very unlikely. This idea will be explored further in Chapter 7 below.

2. For more on how narratives partially construct disease outbreaks, see Briggs and Mantini-Briggs 2007.

3. Guillain–Barré Syndrome is defined by the National Institutes of Health as "a disorder in which the body's immune system attacks part of the peripheral nervous system." The syndrome often develops after a viral infection and is extremely rare in its occurrence. Occasionally, the syndrome can develop in response to vaccinations. See http://www.ninds.nih.gov/disorders/gbs/gbs. htm for a thorough discussion.

4. Controversy erupted in late 2011 when researchers in two prominent labs that study influenza announced they had genetically modified the H5N1 virus into deadlier, more transmissible strains. A temporary moratorium on H5N1 research was called for and implemented in January 2012, as government officials and the scientific community continued to debate the safety and importance of such research. Experts also argued over whether or not such research should be made publicly available in scientific journals such as *Nature* or *Science*. The initial H5N1 papers were temporarily held as the larger research community debated the effects of publication. By early April 2012, the decision to hold the papers was rescinded and the scientific results were published. The entire incident had the effect not only of capturing the public's attention and reinvigorating fears over "bird flu," but of causing a retooling of official policy in relationship to scientific research on potentially dangerous biological agents. See *Science*'s online timeline of the H5N1 controversy for more detail: http://www.sciencemag.org/site/special/h5n1/timeline/index.xhtml.

5. Experts working in public health often shorten influenza virus subtypes to just their "H" numbers. H1N1 is referred to as simply "H1" and H5N1 is truncated to "H5." This practice is common both in Atlanta and in Hong Kong.

5. The Predictable Unpredictability of Viruses and the Concept of "Strategic Uncertainty"

1. Hardt and Negri persuasively argue in their book *Empire* (2001) that an environment of sustained crisis is foundational to the operation of a new type of globalized power structure.

2. My use of "strategic uncertainty" here is distinct from the term as originally coined within economic theory by Van Huyck, Battalio, and Beil (1990). As Donald Moynihan has explained, strategic uncertainty in economic and management theory typically refers to a specific type of uncertainty that "arises because networks contain multiple actors who retain some measure of strategic autonomy, creating uncertainty about what choices they will make." Thus, "strategic" is a qualitative term used to describe the type of uncertainty being experienced by actors in a network, "as the various actors seek to maximize their position in the network but know little about the intentions of other actors." (Moynihan 2008, 354, 356.) Strategic uncertainty as I utilize it here refers instead to the strategic *deployment* of uncertainty, where "strategic" is a descriptive term used in relationship to an actor's intentions when discussing uncertainty. My usage here relates, then, to how uncertainty itself becomes a rhetorical device or narrative tool for retaining scientific authority during the pandemic.

3. I first began thinking about the role of ambiguity in public health after a correspondence with Dr. Linsey McGoey regarding a 2009 workshop she organized at the University of Oxford's Said Business School, entitled "Strategic Unknowns: The Usefulness of Ambiguity and Ignorance in Organizational Life." The conference examined the various political, economic, and social uses of ambiguity and ignorance in a variety of fields and sites. The economic concept I use throughout this chapter, "strategic uncertainty," is in many ways an outgrowth of my engagement with the idea of the "strategic unknown." Ambiguity here is used to refer to the opacity inherent to the

production of scientific information, whereas uncertainty is used to denote an ontological property of the knowledge produced about the virus itself.

4. This chapter originally appeared in the political theory journal *Behemoth*, as part of a special issue looking at new ways of configuring "epidemic order" in public health. I thank the editor of the special issue, Carlo Caduff, and three anonymous peer reviewers for their contributions to the development of the ideas presented here.

5. I do not mean to suggest that uncertainty about the influenza virus or the pandemic itself was wholly manufactured. The public health experts that I interviewed felt that there was indeed much uncertainty about both the virus and the events themselves—especially during the first few months of the pandemic. What I find most interesting—and what I will focus on here—is how they spoke about or deployed that biological uncertainty to positive effect, and how uncertainty was partially managed by transforming it back into certainty about the unpredictability of viruses.

6. The charge was made in an article by *BMJ* features editor Deborah Cohen and investigative journalist Philip Carter, who suggested that the WHO's reputation had been damaged by its lack of transparency and its reluctance to publicly disclose the names of its key scientific advisers on influenza during the pandemic response. Some of these scientists had been shown to have connections with or to have taken payments from pharmaceutical companies responsible for manufacturing not only influenza vaccines, but drugs used in the mitigation of flu (such as Relenza).

6. The Anthropology of Good Information

1. Boyer's ethnography tracks the information overload of journalists—whose job it is not only to "produce content" but also increasingly to contextualize and add analysis to the news. The fatigue and stress caused by these new tasks and by a "faster" information flow mimics what I observed inside the CDC.

2. In 2005, following SARS, the WHO revised its list of reportable infectious diseases and reorganized the categories of disease of international importance or concern. Member nations use this list to craft their own reportable lists. See http://www.cdc.gov/mmwr/PDF/wk/mm5853.pdf for an example of a comprehensive CDC list from 2009.

3. For security purposes, and to protect those I worked with, the names of these countries as well as specific locations of outbreaks, have been omitted.

7. The Heretics of Microbiology

1. In the preface to the seminal 1993 volume *Emerging Viruses*, edited by famed epidemiologist Stephen S. Morse, he reminds his readers that notwithstanding a desire to "anticipate emerging disease, we cannot foretell the future." Instead, Morse argues that the past should be a "valuable guide" from which to deduce possible futures (Morse 1993, viii).

2. Anthropologist Carlo Caduff has written an article (2014) about the difference in opinion between the two main scions of influenza research, Robert Webster and Peter Palese. Dr. Palese's opinions are very similar to those expressed here by Fred Leung.

3. Guan Yi is one of the premier researchers of infectious disease—including influenza—in Hong Kong. His work is often cited by other virologists and epidemiologists working on the subject. He discovered the SARS coronavirus, along with Malik Peiris at HKU, in 2003. Guan Yi is also outspoken in his support of culling chickens and closing wet markets to halt the spread of H5N1. Wet markets in China traditionally sell live animals and fish for consumption. Chinese consumers often prefer this "fresh" meat to the prepackaged variety found in more Western-style supermarkets.

Epilogue

1. My thanks to Stefanie Graeter and Jerry Zee for organizing the 2013 AAA panel entitled "Ethnographies of Exposure." My initial formulation of this concept was a result of their

invitation and prodded me to think through the relationship between ecology and exposure more rigorously.

2. An important aside: Under the rubric of "pandemic humanity" as I've constructed it here, Anna Tsing's focus on global "frictions" (2005) rather than flows might be either reread or reconstituted as social "reassortant events" that produce new cultural forms. Pathography, then, would pay attention to both flow and friction (as friction cannot exist without flow).

REFERENCES

Abbas, M. A. 1997. *Hong Kong: Culture and the Politics of Disappearance*. Minneapolis: University of Minnesota Press.

Adams, Vincanne, Michelle Murphy, and Adele Clarke. 2009. "Anticipation: Technoscience, Life, Affect, Temporality." *Subjectivity* (28): 246–65.

Alcabes, Philip. 2009. *Dread: How Fear and Fantasy Have Fueled Epidemics from the Black Death to Avian Flu*. New York: PublicAffairs.

Altman, Lawrence K. 2009. "Sound the Alarm? A Swine Flu Bind." *New York Times*, April 27.

American Anthropological Association. 1993. *92nd American Anthropological Association Annual Meeting 1993: Cyborg Anthropology*. Washington, DC, 1993.

Anderson, Benedict R. O'G. 1983. *Imagined Communities: Reflections on the Origin and Spread of Nationalism*. London: Verso.

Anderson, Warwick. 2006. *Colonial Pathologies: American Tropical Medicine, Race, and Hygiene in the Philippines*. Durham: Duke University Press.

Arnold, David. 1993. *Colonizing the Body: State Medicine and Epidemic Disease in Nineteenth-century India*. Berkeley: University of California Press.

Artenstein, Andrew W., ed. 2010. *Vaccines: A Biography*. New York: Springer.

Atlani-Duault, Laetitia, and Carl Kendall. 2009. "Influenza, Anthropology, and Global Uncertainties." *Medical Anthropology Quarterly* 28 (3): 207–11.

Bakhtin, M. M. 1981. *The Dialogic Imagination: Four Essays*, edited by Michael Holquist. Austin: University of Texas Press.

Barad, Karen. 1999. "Agential Realism." In Biagioli 1999, 1–11.

Baudrillard, Jean, Sylvère Lotringer, and Ames Hodges. 2010. *The Agony of Power*. Los Angeles: Semiotext(e).

Bauman, Richard, and Charles L. Briggs. 1990. "Poetics and Performances as Critical Perspectives on Language and Social Life." *Annual Review of Anthropology* 19: 59–88.

Bayart, Jean-François. 2005. *The Illusion of Cultural Identity*. London: Hurst.

Bennett, Jane. 2010. *Vibrant Matter: A Political Ecology of Things*. Durham: Duke University Press.

Berlant, Lauren Gail. 2011. *Cruel Optimism*. Durham: Duke University Press.

Bhoumik, Priyasma, and Austin L. Hughes. 2010. "Reassortment of Ancient Neurominidase and Recent Hemagglutinin in Pandemic (H1N1) 2009 Virus." *Emerging Infectious Diseases* 16 (11): 1748–50.

Biagioli, Mario. 1999. *The Science Studies Reader*. New York: Routledge.

Blakely, Debra E. 2003. "Social Construction of Three Influenza Pandemics in the *New York Times*." *Journalism & Mass Communication Quarterly* (80): 884–902.

Boellstorff, Tom. 2008. *Coming of Age in Second Life: An Anthropologist Explores the Virtually Human*. Princeton: Princeton University Press.

Boivin, Nicole. 2010. *Material Cultures, Material Minds: The Impact of Things on Human Thought, Society, and Evolution*. Cambridge: Cambridge University Press.

Bourdieu, Pierre. 2004. *Science of Science and Reflexivity*, trans. Richard Nice. Chicago: University of Chicago Press.

Bowker, Geoffrey C., and Susan Leigh Star. 1999. *Sorting Things Out: Classification and Its Consequences*. Cambridge, Mass.: MIT Press.

Boyer, Dominic. 2005. "The Corporeality of Expertise." *Ethnos: Journal of Anthropology* 70 (2): 243–66.

——. 2013. *The Life Informatic: Newsmaking in the Digital Era*. Ithaca: Cornell University Press.

Bradsher, Keith. 2009. "The Naming of Swine Flu, A Curious Matter." *New York Times*, April 29.

Brandt, Allan M. 1987. *No Magic Bullet: A Social History of Venereal Disease in the United States since 1880*. New York: Oxford University Press.

Briggs, C. L., and M. Nichter. 2009. "Biocommunicability and the Biopolitics of Pandemic Threats." *Medical Anthropology* 28 (3): 189–98.

Briggs, Charles L., and Clara Mantini-Briggs. 2003. *Stories in the Time of Cholera: Racial Profiling during a Medical Nightmare*. Berkeley: University of California Press.

Brockwell-Staats, C., R. G. Webster, and R. J. Webby. 2009. "Diversity of Influenza Viruses in Swine and the Emergence of a Novel Human Pandemic Influenza A (H1N1)." *Influenza and Other Respiratory Viruses* 3 (5): 207–13.

Broor, S., et al. 2012. "Dynamic Patterns of Circulating Seasonal and Pandemic A(H1N1)pdm09 Influenza Viruses from 2007–2010 in and around Delhi, India." PLoS One 7(1):e29129.

Brown, Mark B. 2009. *Science in Democracy: Expertise, Institutions, and Representation*. Cambridge, Mass.: MIT Press.

Caduff, Carlo. Forthcoming. "Pandemic Prophecy: Or, How to Have Faith in Reason." *Current Anthropology.*

Callahan, Gerald N. 2006. *Infection: The Uninvited Universe.* New York: St. Martin's Press.

Callon, Michel. 1999 [1986]. "Some Elements of a Sociology of Translation: Domestication of the Scallops and the Fishermen of St. Brieuc Bay." In Biagioli 1999, 67–83.

Callon, Michel, Pierre Lascoumes, and Yannick Barthe. 2009. *Acting in an Uncertain World: An Essay on Technical Democracy.* Cambridge, Mass.: MIT Press.

Campbell, Brian L. 1985. "Uncertainty as Symbolic Action in Disputes Among Experts." *Social Studies of Science* 15: 429–53.

Carr, E. Summerson. 2010. "Enactments of Expertise." *Annual Review of Anthropology* (39): 17–32.

Carroll, John M. 2007. *A Concise History of Hong Kong.* Lanham: Rowman & Littlefield.

Castells, Manuel. 2010. *The Rise of the Network Society.* Chichester, UK.

Chen, Kuan-Hsing. 2010. *Asia as Method: Toward Deimperialization.* Durham: Duke University Press.

China Daily. 2009a. "Envoy Says Virus Didn't Originate in Mexico." http://www.chinadaily.com.cn/world/2009-04/28/content_7721999.htm.

——. 2009b. "Reports on Disease Origin 'Groundless.'" http://www.chinadaily.com.cn/world/2009-04/30/content_7731551.htm.

Choy, Tim. 2005. "Articulated Knowledges: Environmental Forms after Universality's Demise." *American Anthropologist* 107 (1): 5–18.

Christakis, Nicholas. 2010. "The Hidden Influence of Social Networks." Technology, Entertainment, Design (TED) Conference, http://www.ted.com/talks/nicholas_christakis_the_hidden_influence_of_social_networks.html.

Cohen, Deborah, and Philip Carter. 2010. "WHO and the Pandemic Flu 'Cconspiracies.'" *British Medical Journal* 340:c2912.

Cohen, Jon. 2009a. "Flu Researchers Train Sights on Novel Tricks of Novel H1N1." *Science* 324 (5929): 870–71.

——. 2009b. "Out of Mexico? Scientists Ponder Swine Flu's Origins." *Science* 324 (5928): 700–702.

——. 2009c. "Past Pandemics Provide Mixed Clues to H1N1's Next Moves." *Science* 324 (5930): 996–97.

Cohen, Jon, and Martin Enserink. 2009a. "As Swine Flu Circles Globe, Scientists Grapple with Basic Questions." *Science* 324 (5927): 572–73.

——. 2009b. "Virus of the Year: The Novel H1N1 Influenza." *Science* 326 (5960): 1607.

Coleman, E. Gabriella. 2013. *Coding Freedom: The Ethics and Aesthetics of Hacking.* Princeton: Princeton University Press.

Collins, H. M., and Robert Evans. 2007. *Rethinking Expertise.* Chicago: University of Chicago Press.

Comay, Rebecca. 2000. "Adorno's Siren Song." *New German Critique* (81): 21–48.

Cronon, William. 1992. "A Place for Stories: Nature, History, and Narrative." *Journal of American History* 78 (4): 1347–76.

Crosby, Alfred. 2003. *America's Forgotten Pandemic: The Influenza of 1918.* Cambridge: Cambridge University Press.

Davies, Pete. 2000. *The Devil's Flu: The World's Deadliest Influenza Epidemic and the Scientific Hunt for the Virus That Caused It.* New York: Henry Holt & Co.

Davis, Mike. 2005. *The Monster at Our Door: The Global Threat of Avian Flu.* New York: New Press.

Dawkins, Richard. 1976. *The Selfish Gene.* New York: Oxford University Press.

DeGolyer, Michael E. 2004. "How the Stunning Outbreak of Disease Led to a Stunning Outbreak of Dissent." In Loh 2004, 117–38.

Douglas, Mary. 1966. *Purity and Danger: An Analysis of Concepts of Pollution and Taboo.* London: Routledge & Kegan Paul.

———. 1986. *How Institutions Think.* Syracuse: Syracuse University Press.

Dunn, Elizabeth. 2009. "Standards without Infrastructure." In *Standards and Their Stories: How Quantifying, Classifying, and Formalizing Practices Shape Everyday Life*, edited by Martha Lampland and Susan Leigh Star, 118–21. Ithaca: Cornell University Press.

Durkheim, Emile. 1984 [1893]. *The Division of Labor in Society*, trans. W. D. Halls. New York: Free Press.

Elster, Jon. 1979. *Ulysses and the Sirens: Studies in Rationality and Irrationality.* Cambridge: Cambridge University Press.

Escobar, Arturo. 1994. "Welcome to Cyberia: Notes on the Anthropology of Cyberculture." *Current Anthropology* 35 (3): 211–31.

Esposito, Roberto. 2008. *Bios: Biopolitics and Philosophy.* Minneapolis: University of Minnesota Press.

Evans, Grant, and Siumi Maria Tam. 1997. *Hong Kong: The Anthropology of a Chinese Metropolis.* Honolulu: University of Hawai'i Press.

Ewald, Paul W. 2000. *Plague Time: How Stealth Infections Cause Cancers, Heart Disease, and Other Deadly Ailments.* New York: Free Press.

Fabian, Johannes. 1983. *Time and the Other: How Anthropology Makes Its Object.* New York: Columbia University Press.

Farmer, Paul. 2006. *AIDS and Accusation: Haiti and the Geography of Blame.* Berkeley: University of California Press.

Ferguson, James. 1994. *The Anti-Politics Machine: "Development," Depoliticization, and Bureaucratic Power in Lesotho.* Minneapolis: University of Minnesota Press, 1994.

Finlayson, James Gordon. 2005. *Habermas: A Very Short Introduction.* Oxford: Oxford University Press.

Fischer, Michael M. J., et al. 2008. "Anthropology of/in Circulation: The Future of Open Access and Scholarly Societies." *Cultural Anthropology* 23 (3): 559–88.

Fleck, Ludwik. 1979. *Genesis and Development of a Scientific Fact.* Chicago: University of Chicago Press.

Floridi, Luciano. 2010. *Information: A Very Short Introduction.* Oxford: Oxford University Press.

FluGenome. 2010. "Genotyping Influenza A Viruses with Full Genome Sequences." http://www.flugenome.org.

Fonte, Verona. 2006. *Bird Flu: What To Do.* Berkeley: Iris Arts Press.

Foucault, Michel. 1973. *The Birth of the Clinic; An Archaeology of Medical Perception.* New York: Pantheon Books.

———. 1979. "On Governmentality." *Ideology and Consciousness* (6): 5–21.

———. 1984. *The Foucault Reader*, edited by Paul Rabinow. New York: Pantheon Books.

———. 1988. *The History of Sexuality*, Vol. 3: *The Care of the Self*. New York: Vintage Books.

Fraser, Christophe, et al. 2009. "Pandemic Potential of a Strain of Influenza A (H1N1): Early Findings." *Science* 324: 1557–61.

Fuller, T. L., et al. 2013. "Predicting Hotspots for Influenza Virus Reassortment." *Emerging Infectious Diseases* 19 (4): 581–88.

Gandhi, Leela. 1998. *Postcolonial Theory: A Critical Introduction*. New York: Columbia University Press.

Gardner, Amanda. 2010. "As Swine Flu Fades, Experts Ponder Next Season." Bloomberg Businessweek.

Garfinkel, Harold. 2008. *Toward a Sociological Theory of Information*. Boulder: Paradigm.

Garrett, Laurie. 1994. *The Coming Plague: Newly Emerging Diseases in a World Out of Balance*. New York: Farrar, Straus and Giroux.

———. 2013. "Is This a Pandemic Being Born?" *Foreign Policy*. Blog post (April 1). http://www.foreignpolicy.com/articles/2013/04/01/is_this_a_pandemic_being_born_china_pigs_virus.

Garten, R. J., et al. 2009. "Antigenic and Genetic Characteristics of Swine-origin 2009 A (H1N1) Influenza Viruses Circulating in Humans." *Science* 325 (5937): 197–201.

Gilman, Sander L. 1988. *Disease and Representation: Images of Illness from Madness to AIDS*. Ithaca: Cornell University Press.

Goffman, Erving. 1959. *The Presentation of Self in Everyday Life*. Garden City: Doubleday.

Grady, Denise. 2009. "W.H.O. Gives Virus a Name That's More Scientific and Less Loaded." *New York Times*, April 30.

Greene, Jeffrey. 2006. *The Bird Flu Pandemic: Can It Happen? Will It Happen? How to Protect Yourself and Your Family if It Does*. New York: Thomas Dunne.

Hamilton, Edith. 1963. *Mythology*. New York: Grosset & Dunlap.

Hardt, Michael, and Antonio Negri. 2000. *Empire*. Cambridge, Mass.: Harvard University Press.

Hart, Roger. 1999. "Beyond Science and Civilization: A Post-Needham Critique." *East Asian Science, Technology, and Medicine* (16): 88–114.

Hayden, Cori. 2003. *When Nature Goes Public: The Making and Unmaking of Bioprospecting in Mexico*. Princeton: Princeton University Press.

Hayden, E. C. 2009. "Avian Influenza Aided Readiness for Swine Flu." *Nature* 459 (7248): 756–57.

Helmreich, Stefan. 2009. *Alien Ocean: Anthropological Voyages in Microbial Seas*. Berkeley: University of California Press.

Hilgartner, Stephen. 2000. *Science on Stage: Expert Advice as Public Drama*. Stanford: Stanford University Press.

Ho, Faith. 2006a. *Plague, SARS and the Story of Medicine in Hong Kong*. Hong Kong: Hong Kong University Press.

———. 2006b. *The Silent Protector: A Short Centennial History of Hong Kong's Bacteriological Institute*. Hong Kong: Hong Kong Museum of Medical Sciences.

Ho, Karen Zouwen. 2009. *Liquidated: An Ethnography of Wall Street*. Durham: Duke University Press.

Horkheimer, Max, and Theodor W. Adorno. 2002. *Dialectic of Enlightenment: Philosophical Fragments*, edited by Gunzelin Schmid Noerr. Stanford: Stanford University Press.

Hughes, Richard. 1968. *Hong Kong: Borrowed Place, Borrowed Time*. London: Deutsch.

Institute of Medicine. 1992. *Emerging Infections: Microbial Threats to Health in the United States*. Washington: National Academy Press.

Kelty, Christopher M. 2008. *Two Bits: The Cultural Significance of Free Software*. Durham: Duke University Press.

Kleinman, Arthur. 1980. *Patients and Healers in the Context of Culture: An Exploration of the Borderland between Anthropology, Medicine, and Psychiatry*. Berkeley: University of California Press.

Kleinman, Arthur, and James L. Watson. 2006. *SARS in China: Prelude to Pandemic?* Stanford: Stanford University Press.

Knorr-Cetina, K. 1999. *Epistemic Cultures: How the Sciences Make Knowledge*. Cambridge, Mass.: Harvard University Press.

Kolata, Gina Bari. 1999. *Flu: The Story of the Great Influenza Pandemic of 1918 and the Search for the Virus That Caused It*. New York: Farrar, Straus and Giroux.

Kroeber, Alfred. 1917. "The Superorganic." *American Anthropologist* 19 (2): 163–213.

Lakoff, Andrew, and Stephen J. Collier. 2008. *Biosecurity Interventions: Global Health and Security in Question*. New York: Columbia University Press.

Lampland, Martha, and Susan Leigh Star. 2009. *Standards and Their Stories: How Quantifying, Classifying, and Formalizing Practices Shape Everyday Life*. Ithaca: Cornell University Press.

Latour, Bruno. 1993. *We Have Never Been Modern*. Cambridge, Mass.: Harvard University Press.

———. 2005. *Reassembling the Social: An Introduction to Actor-Network-Theory*. Oxford: Oxford University Press.

Latour, Bruno, and Steve Woolgar. 1979. *Laboratory Life: The Social Construction of Scientific Facts*. Beverly Hills: Sage.

Lau, Alexis. 2004. "The Numbers Trail: What the Data Tells Us." In Loh 2004, 81–94.

Laurel, Brenda, and S. Joy Mountford. 1990. *The Art of Human-Computer Interface Design*. Reading, Mass.: Addison-Wesley.

Leung, Gabriel. 2004. "The Public Health Viewpoint." In Loh 2004, 55–80.

Liu, Xin. 2002. *The Otherness of Self: A Genealogy of the Self in Contemporary China*. Ann Arbor: University of Michigan Press.

Lo, Kwai-Cheung. 2005. *Chinese Face/Off: The Transnational Popular Culture of Hong Kong*. Urbana: University of Illinois Press.

Loh, Christine, ed. 2004. *At the Epicentre: Hong Kong and the SARS Outbreak*. Hong Kong: Hong Kong University Press.

Lowe, Celia. 2010. "Viral Clouds: Becoming H5N1 in Indonesia." *Cultural Anthropology* 25 (4): 625–49.

Lyotard, Jean-François. 1984. *The Postmodern Condition: A Report on Knowledge*. Minneapolis: University of Minnesota Press.

MacPhail, Theresa. 2004. "The Viral Gene: an Undead Metaphor Recoding Life." *Science as Culture* 13 (3): 325–45.

———. 2009. "The Politics of Bird Flu: The Battle over Viral Samples and China's Role in Global Public Health." *Journal of Language and Politics* 8 (3): 456–75.

———. 2010. "A Predictable Unpredictability: The 2009 H1N1 Pandemic and the Concept of 'Strategic Uncertainty' within Global Public Health." *Behemoth* (3): 57–77.

Madsen, Richard. 1995. *China and the American Dream: A Moral Inquiry*. Berkeley: University of California Press.

Maglen, K. 2003. "Politics of Quarantine in the 19th Century." *JAMA* 290 (21): 2873.

Maher, Brendan. 2010. "Swine Flu: Crisis Communicator." *Nature* (463): 150–52.

Malinowski, Bronislaw. 1922. *Argonauts of the Western Pacific*. Long Grove: Waveland Press, Inc.

Margulis, Lynn, and Dorion Sagan. 2002. *Acquiring Genomes: A Theory of the Origins of Species*. New York: Basic Books.

Martin, Emily. 1994. *Flexible Bodies: Tracking Immunity in American Culture from the Days of Polio to the Age of AIDS*. Boston: Beacon Press.

Masco, Joseph. Forthcoming. *The Theater of Operations: Affective Infrastructures of the National Security State*. Durham: Duke University Press.

Matthews, R. E. 1985. "Viral Taxonomy for the Nonvirologist." *Annual Review of Microbiology* 39: 451–74.

Mauss, Marcel. 1954. *The Gift; Forms and Functions of Exchange in Archaic Societies*. Glencoe: Free Press.

McNeil, Donald G. 2009. "In New Theory, Swine Flu Started in Asia, Not Mexico." *New York Times*, June 24.

Michaels, David, and Celeste Monforton. 2005. "Manufacturing Uncertainty: Contested Science and the Protection of the Public's Health and Environment." *American Journal of Public Health* 95 (S1): S39–βS48.

Miller, Vincent. 2011. *Understanding Digital Culture*. Los Angeles: Sage.

Mitchell, Timothy. 2002. *Rule of Experts: Egypt, Techno-politics, Modernity*. Berkeley: University of California Press.

MMWR Weekly. 2009. "Swine Influenza A (H1N1) Infection in Two Children— Southern California, March–April 2009." April 24, http://www.cdc.gov/mmwr/pre view/mmwrhtml/mm5815a5.htm.

Moore, Pete. 2007. *The Little Book of Pandemics: 50 of the World's Most Virulent Plagues and Infectious Diseases*. New York: Collins.

Morens, D. M., and J. K. Taubenberger. 2010. "Historical Thoughts on Influenza Viral Ecosystems, or Behold a Pale Horse, Dead Dogs, Failing Fowl, and Sick Swine." *Influenza and Other Respiratory Viruses* 4 (6): 327–37.

Morse, Stephen S., ed. 1993. *Emerging Viruses*. New York: Oxford University Press.

Morse, Stephen S., and Ann Schluederberg. 1990. "Emerging Viruses: The Evolution of Viruses and Viral Diseases." *Journal of Infectious Diseases* 162: 1–7.

Moynihan, Donald P. 2008. "Learning under Uncertainty: Networks in Crisis Management." *Public Administration Review* 68 (2): 350–65.

Nelson, Nicole, Anna Geltzer, and Stephen Hilgartner. 2008. "Introduction: The Anticipatory State: Making Policy-relevant Knowledge about the Future." *Science and Public Policy* 35 (8): 546–50.

New York Times. 1918. "Revise Timetable in Influenza Fight," October 6.

Oldstone, Michael B. A. 1998. *Viruses, Plagues, and History*. New York: Oxford University Press.

Pinch, Trevor. 1981. "The Sun-Set: The Presentation of Certainty in Scientific Life." *Social Studies of Science* (11): 131–58.

Porter, Dorothy. 1999. *Health, Civilization, and the State: A History of Public Health from Ancient to Modern Times*. London: Routledge.

Potter, C. W. 2001. "A History of Influenza." *Journal of Applied Microbiology* (91): 572–79.

Rabinow, Paul. 1996. *Making PCR: A Story of Biotechnology*. Chicago: University of Chicago Press.

Rheinberger, Hans-Jörg. 2010. *An Epistemology of the Concrete: Twentieth-century Histories of Life*. Durham: Duke University Press.

Riles, Annelise. 2000. *The Network Inside Out*. Ann Arbor: University of Michigan Press.

Rogaski, Ruth. 2004. *Hygienic Modernity: Meanings of Health and Disease in Treaty-Port China*. Berkeley: University of California Press.

Rosen, George. 1958. *A History of Public Health*. New York,: MD Publications.

Rosenberg, Charles E., and Janet Lynne Golden, eds. 1992. *Framing Disease: Studies in Cultural History*. New Brunswick: Rutgers University Press.

Rosenwald, Michael. 2006. "The Flu Hunter." http://www.smithsonianmag.com/science-nature/flu.html.

Romanucci-Ross, Lola. 1977. "The Hierarchy of Resort in Curative Practices: The Admiralty Islands, Melanesia." In *Culture, Disease, and Healing: Studies in Medical Anthropology*, edited by David Landy, 481–86. New York: Macmillan.

Scheper-Hughes, Nancy and Margaret M. Lock. 1987. "The Mindful Body: A Prolegomenon to Future Work in Medical Anthropology." *Medical Anthropology Quarterly* 1 (1): 6–41.

Science. 2009. "Outbreak Ticktock." 324 (22): 700–703.

ScienceDaily. 2009. "Researchers Describe the 90-year Evolution of Swine Flu." http://www.sciencedaily.com/releases/2009/06/090629200641.htm.

Searle, John R. 1995. *The Construction of Social Reality*. New York: Free Press.

Sepkowitz, Kent A. 2009. "Forever Unprepared: The Predictable Unpredictability of Pathogens." *New England Journal of Medicine* 361 (2): 120–21.

Shackley, Simon, and Brian Wynne. 1996. "Representing Uncertainty in Global Climate Change Science and Policy: Boundary-ordering Devices and Authority." *Science, Technology & Human Values* 21 (3): 275–302.

Shapin, Steven, and Simon Schaffer. 1985. *Leviathan and the Air-Pump: Hobbes, Boyle, and the Experimental Life*. Princeton: Princeton University Press.

Shen, Simon. 2008. "Borrowing the Hong Kong Identity for Chinese Diplomacy: Implications of Margaret Chan's World Health Organization Election Campaign." *Pacific Affairs* 81 (3): 361–82.

Silberner, Joanne, and Nell Greenfieldboyce. 2009. "Flu Genes Suggest Virus Not As Deadly As 1918." NPR, May 1. http://www.npr.org/templates/story/story.php?storyId=103678167.

Singer, Merrill. 2009. "Pathogens Gone Wild? Medical Anthropology and the 'Swine Flu' Pandemic." *Medical Anthropology Quarterly* 28 (3): 199–206.

Sipress, Alan. 2009. *The Fatal Strain: On the Trail of Avian Flu and the Coming Pandemic*. New York: Viking.

Spencer, Herbert. 1969 [1876]. *Principles of Sociology*, ed. Stanislav Andreski. London,: Macmillan.

Star, Susan Leigh. 1985. "Scientific Work and Uncertainty." *Social Studies of Science* (15): 391–427.

Star, Susan Leigh, and James R. Griesemer. 1999. "Institutional Ecology, 'Translation,' and Boundary Objects: Amateurs and Professionals in Berkeley's Museum of Vertebrate Zoology, 1907–39." In Biagioli 1999, 505–24.

Stengers, Isabelle. 2000. *The Invention of Modern Science*, trans. Daniel W. Smith. Minneapolis: University of Minnesota Press.

Tamerius, J. D., et al. 2013. "Environmental Predictors of Seasonal Influenza Epidemics across Temperate and Tropical Climates." PLOS Pathogens 9 (3):e1003194.

Taubenberger, Jeffery K., and David M. Morens. 2006. "1918 Influenza: The Mother of All Pandemics." *Emerging Infectious Diseases* 12 (1): 15–22.

Trifonov, V., H. Khiabanian, B. Greenbaum, and R. Rabadan. 2009. "The Origin of the Recent Swine Influenza A (H1N1) Virus Infecting Humans." Euro Surveillance 14 (17):pii = 19193.

Tsang, Thomas H. F. 2009. "The Experience of Hong Kong." In *China's Capacity to Manage Infectious Diseases: Global Implications*, edited by Xiaoqing Lu. Washington: Center for Strategic and International Studies.

Tsing, Anna Lowenhaupt. 2005. *Friction: An Ethnography of Global Connection*. Princeton: Princeton University Press.

Turkle, Sherry. 2011. *Alone Together: Why We Expect More from Technology and Less from Each Other*. New York: Basic Books.

University of Hong Kong. 2008. *From the Plague to New Emerging Diseases: A Chronicle of Pasteurian Research in Hong Kong*. Hong Kong: University Museum and Art Gallery.

UN News Centre. 2010. "Senior UN Health Official Refutes Accusations of Inflating Risk of H1N1 Flu Pandemic," January 25. http://www.un.org/apps/news/story. asp?NewsID=33584&Cr=h1n1&Cr1=#.UyTxQVy6Vu.

Van Huyck, John B., Raymond C. Battalio, and Richard O. Beil. 1990. "Tacit Coordination Games, Strategic Uncertainty, and Coordination Failure." *American Economic Review* 80 (1): 234–48.

Wald, Priscilla. 2008. *Contagious: Cultures, Carriers, and the Outbreak Narrative*. Durham: Duke University Press.

Watts, S. J. 1997. *Epidemics and History: Disease, Power, and Imperialism*. New Haven: Yale University Press.

Webster, Robert G. 1993. "Influenza." In Morse 1993, 37–45.

Webster, Robert. 2013. Web page at St. Jude Children's Research Hospital site. http://www.stjude.org.

Webster, R. G., et al. 1992. "Evolution and Ecology of Influenza A Viruses." *Microbiology Review* 56 (1): 152–79.

Weeks, Linton. 2009. "Swine Flu: Casting Pearls Before H1N1." NPR, May 1. http://www.npr.org/templates/story/story.php?storyId=103702352.

Wittgenstein, Ludwig. 1969. *On Certainty*. New York: Harper.

Woodson, Grattan, and David Jodrey. 2005. The Bird Flu Preparedness Planner: What It Is, How It Spreads, What You Can Do. Deerfield Beach: Health Communications.

World Health Organization. 2005. *WHO Global Influenza Preparedness Plan: The Role of WHO and Recommendations for National Measures before and during Pandemics.* Geneva: World Health Organization.

———. 2010. "The International Response to the Influenza Pandemic: WHO Responds to the Critics." Pandemic (H1N1) 2009 Briefing Note 21. http://www.who.int/csr/disease/swineflu/notes/briefing_20100610/en/.

Yu, H., et al. 2013. "Human Infection with Avian Influenza A H7N9 Virus: An Assessment of Clinical Severity." *The Lancet* 382 (9887): 138–45.

Zimmer, Carl. 2010. "The Ever-Surprising Swine Flu." *Discover*, February 16. http://blogs.discovermagazine.com/loom/2010/02/16/the-ever-surprising-swine-flu/#.UySc7ly6Vuo.

———. 2012. *A Planet of Viruses*. Chicago: University of Chicago Press.